Wendy Satin Rapaport, L

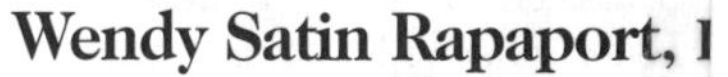

WHEN Diabetes Hits Home

THE WHOLE FAMILY'S GUIDE TO EMOTIONAL HEALTH

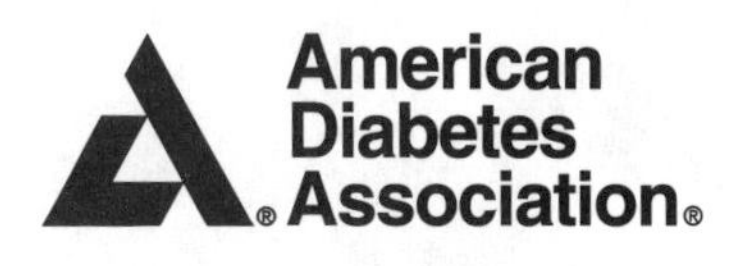

Book Acquisitions: Robert J. Anthony
Editor: Sherrye Landrum
Production Director: Carolyn R. Segree
Production Coordinator: Peggy M. Rote
Desktop Publishing: James Stein Communications
Design: Wickham & Associates, Inc.

Printed in Canada
1 3 5 7 9 10 8 6 4 2

American Diabetes Association
1660 Duke Street
Alexandria, Virginia 22314

Library of Congress Cataloging-in-Publication Data

Rapaport, Wendy Satin, 1947-
When diabetes hits home : the whole family's guide to emotional health / Wendy Satin Rapaport.
p. cm.
ISBN 0-945448-88-0 (pbk.)
1. Diabetes--Psychological aspects--Popular works.
2. Diabetes--Patients--Family relationships. I. Title.
RC660.4.R37 1998
616.4'62--dc21 98-17224
CIP

John T. Devlin, MD
Maine Medical Center
Portland, Maine

Alan M. Jacobson, MD
Joslin Diabetes Center
Boston, Massachusetts

Lois Jovanovic, MD
Sansum Medical Research Foundation
Santa Barbara, California

Carolyn Leontos, RD, CDE, MS
The University of Nevada Cooperative Extension
Las Vegas, Nevada

Peter A. Lodewick, MD
Diabetes Care Center
Birmingham, Alabama

Carol E. Malcom, BSN, CDE
Highline Community Hospital
Seattle, Washington

Wylie McNabb, EdD
The University of Chicago Center for Medical Education and Health Care
Chicago, Illinois

Virginia Peragallo-Dittko, RN, MA, CDE
Winthrop University Hospital
Mineola, New York

Jacqueline Siegel, RN
St. Joseph Hospital
Seattle, Washington

Tim Wysocki, PhD
Nemours Children's Clinic
Jacksonville, Florida

Dedication

It will come as no surprise that I dedicate this book to my family, my treasures:

My mother, Anne Satin Shusterman, who taught me to be sensitive and to care about people, my father, Seymour, and dear stepfather, George. My mom would have been proud of this book second to knowing that I am in a happy marriage. (Do you know the one about the only way to keep a Jewish mother alive is not to get married?)

My sisters and their families: Mary Ellen and Dr. Robert Schwab and Jennifer and Daniel, and Marcia and David Lavipour and Sara, Michael, and Rachel. (I did it in birth order, girls.)

Jim's kids (and mine, too) Dean and Jen and Bruce and Teri and our granddaughter Chelsi, and Jim's sister and brother-in-law, Dr. Irving and Sue Paul.

My dearest husband, Jim, who is a guide, a soul mate, and a love for me. Thank you for all your support with this book. Until the cure, I shall love you to health. (That goes for you, too, M.E.)

A Diabetes Disaster

by Charlotte "Teddie" Yohay

Out of sight, out of mind
How can kids be so unkind?
All the work drives me mad,
My friends are gone,
Now I'm sad.
I'm not there, so I'm forgotten.
Who thought my friends could be so rotten?
I'm not the only one who's insane,
My mom claims she'll go on cocaine.
Then my dad could help her out,
But all he does is scream and shout!
"Why does she get all the attention?"
my sister says with recollection.
What "pricks" these shots can be,
But thanks to them, I'm able to see.
Every time I start to cough...
"Will someone turn that meter off?"
I can't go to school today. Oh
I wish this disease would go away!
"Because of this, your life will be great!"
My mom always says at 8.
I'm sure she's right,
But it's hard to believe
Because of all the shots I receive.
G-d this sucks
Don't you agree,
It's starting to eat away at me.
I miss my friends,
I miss the fun.
Please G-d, show me the sun.
This sounds like a Raffi song,
Me and my dad...
We don't get along.
If we did,
It would be fun.
I love my dad,
But he doesn't know it.
Maybe because I don't show it.
He gets on my nerves, but that's okay.
All parents do in a way.
Hey, my life's not that bad,
Maybe I shouldn't be so sad.
I should get upset sometimes.
No, that wouldn't be a crime.
Once in a while would be okay,
Just as long as it's not every day.
This anxiety is killing me,
I wish someone would set me free!
My mom tried,
But I didn't heed her warning,
That's why I feel so lousy this morning.
I will go to school tomorrow,
Even if I remain in sorrow.
Soon I will be fourteen,
Then I'll become a Beauty Queen.
This disease won't hold me back.
Watch out life,
I will attack.
Tonight I will hit the sack,
Then tomorrow, watch out school,
I'm BACK!

Contents

Acknowledgments

Special mention goes to the Diabetes Research Institute, University of Miami Medical School, for being my home away from home for 20 years. Hats off to the Scientific Director Emeritus, Daniel Mintz, MD.

Thanks and respect to all the patients with whom I have worked, and to that special patient "group" who grew up with me. It has been an honor to know all of you.

I thank my professional colleagues who have also been friends through the years. I begin with Jay Skyler, MD, the finest mentor, colleague, and friend. Ron Goldberg, MD, you are the prince of compassion. Special recognition goes to my cherished mentors, Gary Kleiman and Lisa Schwarz. These are the many other wonderful people I've known and worked with the longest—doctors Lester Baker, Alex Rabinovitch, Rudolpho Alejandro, Michael Reeves, Camillo Leslie, Luigi Meninghini, Annette La Greca, Osa Nyman, Robin Nemery, Paul Jellinger, Jorge Caycedo, Evan Katz, Joan MacCracken, and Leonard Levy, and Debbie Seigler, Denny Skyler, Ilene Lasky Klein, Roberta Stone, Della Matheson,

Gwen Enfield, Lisa Rafkin Mervis, Aleida Saenz, Pat Stenger, and Maureen Murray. Much appreciation to the light around the office, Norma Peck. And thanks for the fun and energy and love from Sally, Martha, Violeta, Rosalyn, Mercy, Dinorah, Iliana, and Aimée.

Love and thanks go to these special people for editing individual chapters: Dr. Barbara Stern, Marcia and David Lavipour, Mary Ellen Schwab, Jennifer Schwab, Daniel Schwab, Debbie Singer, Dr. Jorge Caycedo, Noreen Hall Papatheodorou, Rick Record, Gary Kleiman, Chris McAliley, Henny Goldstein, Maureen Murray, Suzanne Wolfson, Lisa Schwarz, Gayle Portnow, Gloria Rothstein, Barbara Singer, the writers group of Midcoast Maine, and Rhoda and Bill Matson.

A special spot for Suzanne. Lots of love and hope to my "kids," Debbie, Edricka, and Pam. Much love to Suzanne Pallot and Mary High.

To my editor, Sherrye Landrum, who has given me confidence and good advice. To my soul-sister and fellow psychologist, Sandy Bernstein, who read every page and breathed life into me, not to mention good grammar and good taste. Thank you for your brilliance, humility, and generosity.

Thanks to Rebecca Taylor Cohen for painstakingly making red pen corrections look like love through my entire book. Thank you for your continuing friendship.

In memory of some very special people: Adrienne Keller, a dear friend; Bernard Deas; and Denise Ingeneiri.

Introduction

As a social worker and psychologist specializing in individual, family, and group therapy for patients with diabetes for 20 years, I am impressed with the wisdom, grace, and courage that my patients have displayed. In this book, I share some of what I've learned from them in the hopes of relieving the isolation that you and your family may feel. Although it merely scratches the surface of the emotional aspects of living with diabetes, I hope that this book can be helpful to you. Share chapters of it with your family members and friends so you can help each other. You may return to other chapters as your life changes.

In 1988 my experience with diabetes broadened. I became the spouse of a person with type 2 diabetes. Imagine living with your own personal psychologist, invested in modifying your behavior...a dream or a nightmare? There is a real art to giving support without trying to control the other person.

I wrote this book for you, your family, and for your interactions together. It is obvious to me in working with people with type 1 and type 2 diabetes and their families, that when you receive the right kind of support, your emotional adjustment to diabetes is smoother, which leads you to take better care of yourself.

It is difficult enough to control diabetes. It can seem overwhelming also to try to control the feelings and behaviors of others concerning your diabetes. But the feelings and behaviors of others significantly affect how you feel (and behave) about yourself and about taking care of your diabetes.

We all want to learn effective ways to support each other. Together, families can combat the potential casualties caused by the stress of a chronic illness—worry turned into nagging, critical behavior; sibling rivalry turning into guilt, depression, or behavior problems; or the couple's imbalance of feelings and responsibility turning into marital discord. Identifying and dealing with problems can be a great asset to the mental and physical health of the whole family. So, here's to your health, one and all.

> The stories I tell of people and their families are not about real individuals. They are created from composites of many people I have worked with over the years. While people are unique and individual, many situations may sound similar to yours.
>
> Please discuss any changes to your medical regimen with your health care team before making those changes.

For You, the Person with Diabetes

Every time Cassandra, age 17, skipped her insulin shot, she felt an immediate sense of smug satisfaction. Hours later, with regret, guilt, high blood sugar, nausea, and the inability to sleep through the night, she suffered the consequences of her actions. The way she chose to express her hostility seemed to backfire painfully. To Cassandra, it felt like she was being punished twice for the same crime. She thought her crime was having diabetes in the first place.

For years, she silently battled with anxiety and anger over the diagnosis. At the same time, her father withdrew, upsetting her even more. He felt guilty about his family history of diabetes. To compensate for her husband's behavior, Cassandra's mother intensified her attempts to control the diabetes, further inciting Cassandra's anger. Finally, Cassandra despaired because her siblings were jealous of all the attention she got from their mother, and they rejected her.

Cassandra *was* on to something. She needed ways to express her anger, fear, and loneliness. The key was her "silent" battle. She desperately wanted to feel in control of her life and to understand more fully why diabetes had changed the way she felt about herself and how her family treated her. These changes hurt her. The hurt led to anger. Hurt, frustrated, and angry, she tried to rebel against the diabetes. Cassandra got into trouble with the way she chose to express her rebellion and confusion—by not taking her shots. She would have been happier and healthier talking out her hurts, sadness, and disappointments rather than acting them out by behavior that hurt her.

Finally, Cassandra talked to me, a psychologist specializing in the adjustment to diabetes. She began to save not only her own life, both physically and emotionally, but also the life of her family. The time they all spent in emotional pain seems so wasteful to them now. Cassandra realized that the issues of how a family works together—for example, too little or too much involvement—were the same as those her peers were complaining about. Her diabetes only intensified the normal struggles of teenage life and relationships.

Unfortunately, people almost always make their choices *silently* about how to feel, react, and behave. This is because most of us are not conscious of the choices we are making. We think things just happen to us without realizing how our habits of behaving or reacting are part of the things that happen. Usually, we focus on ourselves as victims or on what the other person is doing wrong. We need to focus on the power we have to change our feelings, thoughts, and behavior. This is what leads to change in the situation and the relationship.

THE WHOLE FAMILY IS INVOLVED

Like it or not, diabetes is a family disease and has enormous impact on each family member's self-esteem and behavior.

In Cassandra's case, her father's neglect made her feel as though she had disappointed him. She began to devalue herself. When Cassandra's father understood this, he was shocked by her interpretation. He had viewed her diabetes as *his* fault, *his* failure. He felt helpless that he could only watch and not control the disease. He was ashamed that he could not protect her and keep her safe. Cassandra hated to see her father's pain but was relieved to realize that his shame was not about her. When the members of a family understand each other's feelings, they can communicate better and support each other through good times and bad.

Sandy is a 50-year-old dietitian who has had type 2 diabetes for 10 years. She was referred by another member of the medical team, a physician who was feeling frustrated and unable to help her. For years, without any success, he had urged her to take insulin in addition to oral medication to control her diabetes.

In psychotherapy, Sandy had a chance to sort out why she resisted the information—much of which she already knew professionally—about how to take better care of herself. Whereas she had many feelings about what taking insulin meant to her, Sandy spoke earnestly of her shame about being fat, at bringing the diabetes on herself, and at having to take insulin. She felt so embarrassed that she insisted the team must never tell her physician husband that she required insulin. She was worried that he would say that she brought it on herself and would constantly watch her and put her down. She said the thought of his disdain for her would often trigger some of her eating binges. Whether she was accurate or not about her husband's possible response, it was clear that Sandy felt guilty and saddened and perhaps she projected her feelings—assumed that her feelings were his—onto her husband. Again, her battle was silent.

Sandy and her husband needed more information. For example, thin people can also require insulin, because it is the pancreas that is failing, not the person. They needed support, too. When she finally allowed her husband to come in, he spoke of his failure to help her stay healthy and safe—especially troublesome because he was a physician. He was not ashamed of her; he was ashamed of himself for not comforting her, not being able to fix her, and not controlling her diabetes. He was angry at himself, not just her, when she began to overeat. So it was his resentment of his own inadequacy that appeared to her as antagonism. He was also anxious about her future and did not want to be deprived of his lifelong partner.

Therapy brought about a breakthrough for both of them. After the emotional groundwork was done, Sandy could see what he wanted to give her, felt his love, and began to view her own feelings honestly. She saw herself and her diabetes in a more realistic and positive light. He felt a greater peace about actually being able to help her. His outlook was more realistic, too. The wall that had grown between them began to fade. Their relationship could improve and so could her relationship with diabetes.

Although Cassandra and Sandy are different in age, type of diabetes, religion, race, and marital status, they are similar in their personal feelings about themselves, diabetes, and their family interactions. Once they became conscious of their feelings, they could change and begin to help themselves. Over and over, we see that when you change your view of yourself and your diabetes, you can improve your physical health.

HELPING OR HASSLING?

What about you? Are you ready to focus on you, your feelings, and reactions? It's time to break the silence.

Why don't you really want your family to know too much about your diabetes? Are you worried they'll

- follow you around, probing, correcting, hassling, criticizing?
- worry too much?
- abandon you or be indifferent?

There are many good reasons your family should know as much as you do about your diabetes. You'll have someone

- to give you support. (Especially if they learn to give it in a helpful way.)
- to come up with new ideas or alternative actions to take.
- who can take over for you when you need them.

> **Question:** Can independence, self-care, and family support really occur all at the same time?
>
> **Answer:** Yes. In fact, people usually take better care of themselves when they get the right kind of family support—the kind that respects your dignity and independence.

RESPECT FOR YOURSELF

Your concerns about family involvement—especially overinvolvement and control—are real. Creating a balance in relationships is a problem for us all, even without the extra stress that diabetes can add to the mix. Sometimes we submerge our feelings and needs to meet the feelings and needs of another. A common name for this type of imbalance in relationships is *co-dependence*. In the long run, it does not help anyone to conceal your feelings and problems from the family.

The goal of this book is to give you successful methods for creating *interdependent* relationships, where each person is respected as an individual. The case studies I use are composites of real people learning to live with diabetes. The skills you learn can be used by anyone, with or without diabetes, to create and maintain balanced and close relationships.

This chapter is about the first step, recognizing and expressing feelings—your own and those of your family. When you have a negative feeling, you can learn how to **reframe** it—to see it in a different way. This is a very powerful action. It frees you to see the whole situation differently and almost always leads to better communication within the family. This knowledge can change your life, giving you more personal power, more energy, and more loving support from others.

RESPECT FOR EACH ONE

Intrusive families usually are well meaning and have good intentions. Their words may be harmless, but it's how you perceive the words that can hurt you. Create a neutral ground with them where you can look at their intention and how the interaction feels to each of you. What matters is the timing. Don't talk when you are frustrated and angry. Just as we don't speak with our mouths full, we should not speak when our hearts are full of rage and frustration.

Now think about it. What's behind their intrusion? *Empathy? Concern? Fear? Worry? Personal failure? Overreaction? Guilt? Sadness? Anxiety? Hostility? Pity? Burn out?*

Try to look at the situation through their eyes. Whatever their motives, some will result in behavior that helps you, some won't. But until they recognize their own motives, can you try to give your family the benefit of the doubt? (Don't worry if you don't feel like doing that yet.) In time, you will be able to accept the feelings of your family and try to hear the real message. It may help to realize that they are not doubting you as a person. They are just trying to be involved with managing the diabetes while coping with their own difficult emotions about what diabetes means to them and to you. It will take time to accept your own feelings and move to understanding your family's feelings. They're in the same position. That's why the first step may be to let them know how badly you feel inside.

Unfortunately, the natural response to diabetes itself, or to family members who seem intrusive in your care, can isolate you emotionally and end up being bad for your health. Do the following statements sound familiar?

- **Loneliness:** There's no one to talk to who understands me.
- **Secrecy:** I'm not sharing anything. I don't want any criticism.
- **Denial:** I'm not bothering with it. If I don't think about it, it's not there.
- **Shame:** I'm embarrassed about having it and the way I handle it.
- **Rebellion:** Every time I eat something, I feel content that I'm getting you back for all of your criticism and for the fact of even having diabetes.
- **Anger:** Why me? Mind your own business.
- **Guilt:** I do deserve this.

FEELING YOUR WAY TO BETTER HEALTH

Many people ultimately do handle their diabetes very well both personally (how they feel about it) and technically (how they take care of it). Most people go through at least one period of being stuck or overwhelmed.

It is always a challenge to make peace with diabetes—one that your family has to be a part of. The difficult feelings are normal and part of the process of adjusting to diabetes. The **positive** feelings—respect for your own resiliency, pride in your ability to accept a challenge, amazement at your discipline and self-control, pleasure in your character, power in overcoming despair—are just as normal.

Your goal: Make peace with it. Work on the relationship you have with diabetes. It changes at different stages of life—when you're going to school, getting married, having children, retiring—and depends on your age and whether you have type 1 or type 2 diabetes. Your relationship can also change with the length of time you and diabetes have been together. It will be different and evolve over time after the diagnosis as you deal with the day-to-day unchanging nature of diabetes. It will change again as you deal with potential or real medical complications.

If you want to be more comfortable in your own life, improve your skills in relating to your family, and make a healthy adjustment to diabetes, you need to take the following steps:

1. **Recognize** your own feelings.
2. **Recognize** your family's feelings.
3. Learn to **reframe** your way of listening and speaking.
4. Develop an **interaction plan** that satisfies your and your family's needs.

It's too hard to do diabetes alone. The best kind of interaction brings you closer to your family and closer to your targets in diabetes.

RECOGNIZE YOUR OWN FEELINGS

It's important to know yourself, whether or not you have diabetes. (That doesn't mean only knowing what you like to eat or whether you prefer walking to swimming.) This knowing should go from daily feelings—frustration, contentment—to your general point of view about life. This is actually a life task of every human being. However, to adjust to diabetes, you are challenged to find out specifically what diabetes means to you, grieve about it, and then adapt. You have to respect and accept the difficult and negative emotions that come from having diabetes because they won't go away until you do.

Simon was 50. He had spent 40 years living with diabetes. He was completely healthy except for what he thought was a complication of diabetes—sexual dysfunction. After a thorough medical and psychological evaluation, Simon learned that his impotence was psychological. The news was a relief to him and a great frustration.

- *When Simon was 18, thinking of college, but believing he probably wouldn't live a long life because of his diabetes, he said, "why bother?"*
- *When Simon got married, and the ordinary strains of marriage were being worked out, using the same pessimistic philosophy, he said, "why bother?"*
- *When Simon's business began to fail, and he should have borrowed money to revitalize and save it, he said, "why bother?"*

Now, Simon was bothered. He was depressed and angry that none of the complications he'd expected had occurred. The fear of them had changed the way he lived his life. He had wasted it. While waiting for complications to happen, he had not put enough energy into making his life happy, productive, and healthy.

All the stories of people with diabetes underscore your need to know where you stand with diabetes—philosophically and pragmatically. What is your philosophy? *Do you believe you are alive and well? Self-respecting? Deserving? Challenged? As good as the next person? Better? Living a normal life, even with tremendous "behind-the-scenes" efforts? Do you think this is your cross to bear, or do you focus on more difficult feelings like rage and depression?*

How does your philosophy translate into actions? *Do you feel you deserve as much as everyone else and can therefore assert yourself—about anything—to family, friends, waiters, or doctors? Can you tell your mother-in-law that you appreciate her interest but she's doesn't need to watch what you eat? Can you send back the salad and get another with dressing on the side this time? Can you tell the doctor why you don't want to test your blood sugar at work?* The process in this book is to get a hold on your feelings and then your actions. Becoming aware of how you feel and how it shows up in your behavior is very necessary for your emotional and physical health.

Sometimes cycling through the whole gamut of emotions is necessary. The trick is to keep going until you get to the positive feelings.

We are all different—unique—that's why there are no wrong answers, just answers that fit each person. The questions in the box "Know Your Feelings" should stimulate your awareness of potential problems and possible feelings and your reactions to them. It is important for you to find something positive for yourself in diabetes.

KNOW YOUR FEELINGS

Physical

1. When your body responds to high or low blood sugar, you might feel
   a) out of control
   b) moody
   c) depressed
   d) tired
   e) accepting
   f) other

Psychological

2. If you have many episodes of high or low blood sugar, you might feel
   a) guilty, depressed, ashamed
   b) frustrated, resentful
   c) fearful
   d) dependent/isolated
   e) accepting
   f) other

Adherence (following through on diabetes self-care)

3. The pressure of taking care of yourself. When you ask yourself, "Have I done enough," you might feel
   a) trapped, vacationless
   b) bored, indifferent
   c) overwhelmed
   d) lonely
   e) accepting
   f) other

continued

Family

4. If your family monitors your diabetes, you might feel
   - a) supported, comforted
   - b) jealous
   - c) rebellious
   - d) resentful
   - e) accepting
   - f) other

Burnout

5. When you reach burnout with your diabetes, you might feel
   - a) enough is enough
   - b) exhausted
   - c) next, please (frustrated but with a sense of humor?)
   - d) Vacation-impaired
   - e) Accepting
   - f) other

Future

6. When you have fears for the future, you might feel
   - a) anxious
   - b) intimidated
   - c) increasing denial
   - d) increasingly daring
   - e) accepting
   - f) other

RECOGNIZE YOUR FAMILY'S FEELINGS

You should understand your own feelings thoroughly before you attend to those of others. You do not have to be kind and thoughtful right away, but considering them will make your life easier. When you are ready, reflect on what your family might feel about diabetes by answering the questions in the box "How Does Your Family Feel?"

Your family's response can and will change over time just as yours does and will.

HOW DOES YOUR FAMILY FEEL?

Physical

1. Whenever you have high or low blood sugar, your family might feel
   - a) guilty or scared
   - b) critical, judgmental
   - c) watchful
   - d) doting
   - e) understanding, respectful
   - f) other

Psychological

2. If you have many episodes of high or low blood sugar, your family might feel
   - a) sensitive
   - b) worried
   - c) frustrated
   - d) resentful
   - e) understanding
   - f) other

Adherence

3. When they watch how you take care of yourself, your family might feel
   - a) saddened
   - b) controlling
   - c) angry
   - d) guilty
   - e) understanding
   - f) other

continued

Family

4. When they are "monitoring" your diabetes, your family might feel
   a) burdened
   b) happy to share
   c) inadequate
   d) relieved to share burden
   e) understanding of your feelings
   f) other

Burnout

5. When you reach burnout with diabetes, your family might feel
   a) responsible and angry
   b) cheerleading, motivating
   c) detective efforts are called for
   d) responsible and distancing
   e) understanding
   f) other

Future

6. When confronted by fears for your future, your family might feel
   a) anxious
   b) intimidated
   c) increasing denial
   d) depressed
   e) understanding
   f) other

POSITIVE REFRAMING

What is positive reframing? Reframing means changing the way you look at things. You can change your perception by getting new information or looking at the "facts" in a different way. You are mentally moving the picture frame around to see more of the picture. You may think something is negative until you look at other sides of the situation. For example:

Your spouse yells: You do nothing to help yourself.
Your automatic reaction might be: You always criticize me. You don't understand. You don't love me. I hate you.

Your perception is that he is attacking you. With reframing, your spouse is still yelling, but you can hear and respond differently. First, acknowledge your "ouch" feeling. Then move on to thoughts that will help you feel a new way. He does care about you, and he's worried for your safety.

Your reframed response: You're yelling at me. It sounds critical and angry. I know you're worried and afraid for me because you love me. I don't need to be angry back. I do wish you could stop.

Or, try to understand your spouse's motivation.

You might say: I'm trying to understand why you're yelling. You are a perfectionist, and it must be hard for you to give me credit for all the work I do, especially when it doesn't turn out perfectly.

By giving yourself time to understand and make these comments, you may avoid a fight and receive better help from your family and friends. And feel better about yourself.

Positive reframing is not dishonest or a denial of your own feelings. It is the positive action to take after you acknowledge your feelings. Make sure you take enough time to recognize the feeling you are having. Feelings are neither good nor bad. And they pass. When you let go of a feeling, then you can reframe the way you think about the situation. Before you get into a situation that needs reframing, think of things to calm yourself down. Take ten deep breaths. Release the need to respond immediately. The box "Positive Reframing" provides examples of how to positively reframe your feelings and thoughts.

POSITIVE REFRAMING

1. Your blood sugar levels are high because you ate too much.
   Feelings or thoughts: Frustrated. Overwhelmed. Self-blaming.
   Reframe: I'm normal, not perfect. They'll come down.
2. You have no idea why your blood sugar levels are high.
   Feelings or thoughts: I give up. I can't do it.
   Reframe: Sometimes blood sugar levels make no sense. It's okay. I don't have to understand everything. I just need to get them down.
3. Your blood sugar level went low because you didn't stop for lunch.
   Feelings or thoughts: I screw up all the time. I'm no good.
   Reframe: I'm normal, not perfect. Next time I'll prioritize better and take time to feed myself.
4. You resent having to exercise.
   Feelings or thoughts: No one else is under the pressure I am. Life is unfair.
   Reframe: Well, people without diabetes have to exercise, too. I'm a step ahead.
5. You're thinking of canceling your doctor's appointment because your blood sugar levels are high.
   Feelings or thoughts: Intimidated. Ashamed.
   Reframe: We'll both have to accept that I've burned out. This happens with a chronic disease. Maybe s/he can inspire me with some new ideas.

In a sense, each of us can be our own spin doctors, changing the way we choose to see the world and our place in it. This can lead to new behaviors and living in a way that reflects your new point of view.

There are many ways to respond in a situation. The following example has three. The first two responses are normal but don't really get you anywhere. They are aggressive or passive. The assertive response is an example of positive reframing. You can clearly see how feelings lead to healthy or poor behaviors. You can also see that inserting some time to think between your feelings and your behavior can change the outcome.

Your father says: "I'm sick of you never taking care of yourself."

Natural Negative–Aggressive
Feelings: Angry, defensive
Response: "You are the reason I don't."
Behavior: Overeat, don't take enough insulin, skip blood testing, have high blood sugar
Outcome: Angry and diabetes out of control

Natural Negative–Passive
Feelings: Guilty, burdensome
Response: "I wish I were dead and out of the way."
Behavior: Under-eat, skip blood testing, have low blood sugar
Outcome: Depressed and diabetes out of control

continued

Positive Reframe
Feelings: Angry, guilty (note, these are the same as before)
Now you *insert* these steps:
1. Stay with these feelings.
2. Take 10 deep breaths, relax.
3. Calmly search for new ways to look at what's going on.
   - Why did he say that? He is worried, anxious, and doesn't know how to motivate me but feels that he should.
   - How else can I look at it? I can appreciate those feelings. Those are my sentiments about myself, too! My Dad is expressing my sentiments for me. I need to help us both get back on track. Diabetes is a pain, to say the least. I hate diabetes, not my Dad. I guess we both hate it.

Response: "That makes two of us. Diabetes seems to burden you just as much as it does me."
Behavior: Seek help from support groups and the health care team.
Outcome: Feel relieved and supported. Start taking action.

Is this beginning to make sense? You can have feelings. You can also have control over your feelings. Add some compassion for yourself and others and voilá. You get control over your behavior. Influence over your family. Control over your diabetes. It seems like hard work. At the beginning it is, but thinking positively can become almost automatic with practice.

The following are more examples of **feelings** that are triggered by what seem to be intrusions by family members. Sometimes, of course, a lot of breathing and thought need to be inserted between your feelings and your reactions.

MORE REFRAMED RESPONSES

Nagging: "Don't forget to bring a snack with you."
Your feeling: Put down again, never trusted.
Insert: Breathe, add compassion, think.
Reframed reaction: "Thanks for being supportive. Diabetes is a pain to do alone. I sometimes do forget."

Repetitive: "Did you test?"
Your feeling: Challenged, angry, hurt.
Insert: Breathe, add compassion, think.
Reframed reaction: "Thanks for reminding me. I'm lucky to have you on my side."

Critical: "Can't you control it any better than that?"
Your feeling: Self-doubt, Resentment
Insert: Breathe, add compassion, think.
Reframed reaction: "I'm frustrated by trying to be perfect, too."

Angry: "I'm sick of your overeating."
Your feeling: I have to deal with my own feelings of failure *and* your annoyance.
Insert: Breathe, add compassion, think.
Reframed reaction: "That makes two of us. It's definitely difficult to always be in control."

Controlling: "Don't you think that's enough food now, dear?"
Your feeling: Embarrassed, guilty, angry.
Insert: Breathe, add compassion, think.
Reframed reaction: "Thanks for reminding me. Could you say it in a less condescending way though? I know you want to help."

Rejecting: "I can't be bothered with you."
Your feeling: Rejected, disappointed, hurt.
Insert: Breathe, add compassion, think.
Reframed reaction: "Relax. It's *my* diabetes. I do appreciate your help when you give me some."

Demeaning: "Couldn't control what you ate again? You don't do anything for yourself."
Your feeling: Anger at judgmental, controlling person.
Insert: Breathe, add compassion, think.
Reframed reaction: "I see you get just as frustrated as I do. I try to control my food. I would like it if you tried to control giving out criticism." (This is a time to be assertive.)

Hovering: "Shouldn't you test now? You don't look well."
Your feeling: Shame. Can't even know my own reaction first.
Insert: Breathe, add compassion, think.
Reframed reaction: "We're close; you know me well. You may notice my reactions before I do."

Pitying: "I'll take care of that. Don't worry. Go lie down."
Your feeling: Handicapped, dependent.
Insert: Breathe, add compassion, think.
Reframed reaction: "No, don't *you* worry. I'm a lot hardier than I look. I'll be fine in a few minutes."

The following examples point out how families can learn to ask questions and make suggestions to get a more positive response from you. Notice that feelings can lead to healthy or poor behaviors. (Change the interactions to fit your age group.) The last one or two answers are reframed efforts at communicating on both sides. Appreciate that your family's comments, even when well intentioned and generous, can still trigger negative feelings in you. You are in charge of those feelings.

1. You are crying, whining over having to take a shot before dinner. You're sick of your diabetes. (You don't have to be a child to whine.)

Your mom/dad/spouse says: "Oh honey, if I could take it for you, I would." (Well-meaning attempt to be soothing.)

You feel: Annoyed. It's *your* sadness.

You say: "Your guilt is just adding to my problems. You being nice can't take it away."

Your mom/dad/spouse says: "It could be worse. Didn't you see the people with cancer in the office?"

You feel: Annoyed, also appreciative of perspective.

You say: "Can't I legitimately be sick of this?" (Good helpful question even if said with hostility.)

Your mom/dad/spouse says: "Take your shot now! We'll talk after you do."

You feel: Relieved at being given direction.

You say: "Yes, sir! And thanks, General!" (Humor always helps.)

Your mom/dad/spouse says: "You're crying and cranky. Your blood sugar must be low."

You feel: Relieved by description. Annoyed that everything is about diabetes.

You say: "Do you really think every feeling is about diabetes?"

Your mom/dad/spouse says: "You seem so unhappy. Do you feel like talking a little bit?"

You feel: Appreciative of opportunity to ventilate and complain.

You say: "Thanks, I'm feeling so down."

2. There was a party at school/work, and you ate just as many cookies as everyone else. Your blood sugar reflects it.

Your mom/dad/spouse says: "Do I need to police you at school/work, too, so you won't over-eat?"

You feel: Guilty, resentful, inadequate, and with no intention of improving.

You say: "Right! Get a uniform." (Sarcastic)

Your mom/dad/spouse says: "You don't seem to have any self-control."

You feel: Put down, depressed, disinterested.

You say: "Like mother, like daughter." (ouch)

Your mom/dad/spouse says: "With those high blood sugar levels and bad mood, you'll ruin everyone's day."

You feel: Guilty, depressed, and a little angry.

You say: "So it's not *your* turn this time to ruin it." (Now that's hostility!)

Your mom/dad/spouse says: "Would you like to talk about planning ahead regarding school/work food issues, to avoid the high blood sugar level?"

You feel: Supported, optimistic, effective.

You say: "Great idea!"

Your mom/dad/spouse says: "What are your thoughts and feelings about your blood sugar level?" (How it got there and what to do.)

You feel: Independent, self-critical, hopeful.

You say: "I'm glad you're interested. I hate thinking alone. Diabetes is so hard."

3. Your brother (any age) is stuffing himself with joyous abandon after work or school; you (who have diabetes) join him.

He says: "Stop. You shouldn't be eating so much."

You feel: Resentful, angry.

You say: "Stop. You shouldn't be talking so much."

He says: "I'll love telling on you."

You feel: Revengeful.

You say: "I'll get you back. I'll tell mom/your wife about those magazines in your drawer."

He says: "Don't eat in front of me. It makes me feel guilty."

You feel: Guilty, manipulated, jealous.

You say: "Perfect! Now we both feel bad."

He says: "I've always been impressed that you have better habits than I do."

You feel: Thankful, appreciative of support.

You say: "It is incredibly tough. What a thoughtful brother you are to say that."

4. At dinner, you reach for a second helping of rice. Your father says to your mother, "Can he have that?"

Your mother says: "If you'd come to the appointments with us, you'd know."

You feel: Guilty. Are you causing another fight? Resentful. Dad knows nothing.

You say: "Mom don't pick on Dad. It's my fault."

Your mother says: "Don't put the responsibility on me."

You feel: Anxious. They might fight over your diabetes, again.

You say: "Dad, don't pick on Mom. It's my fault."

Your mother says: "I can't stop her."

You feel: Like an object, and a failed one, at that.

You say: "Stop. It's my fault. I hate being a referee. (And you shouldn't have to be one!)

Your mother says: "Would you find it helpful if your dad and I work with you on portions?"

You feel: Relieved. You'd like Dad to know more. Actually, you feel that you could use some help.

You say: "Perfect. I like it when you both help and when we're all close. I do want you to know I planned ahead for my second portion with exercise and insulin."

DEVELOPING AN INTERACTION PLAN

We need to give and receive support from each other through the everyday hassles and tensions, the negative stuff that we take for granted. (And you thought we only took positive things for granted.) Unfortunately in diabetes, regular interactions often involve anger, annoyance, and impatience with ourselves and with others. A plan for interacting with the people in your life can help you get through the day more smoothly.

As you saw in the preceding examples, you meet issues in every interaction with family, friends, and co-workers that can help you or put up roadblocks for you. The issues revolve around

- feelings
- adherence to diabetes management (lifestyle, food, exercise, and medication)
- independence and self-esteem
- personality factors (yours, mine, and ours)

An interaction plan helps you be ready to handle the issues that are likely to come up. A plan helps you feel calm and competent, and goes a long way toward relieving stress and keeping your blood sugar under control.

You're out to dinner at a restaurant with your family. You order a high-fat, high-sugar, high-calorie dessert. Your family (mom/dad/spouse/kids) says, "Are you sure you want that? I think you've eaten quite a bit already."

You **feel:** Annoyed.
You **breathe** (5 deep breaths).
You **think** about what **they** might be feeling:

- protective of you
- worried about you
- guilty that it was their idea to eat out
- annoyed that your high blood sugar will leave you feeling irritable later

You say to yourself: "I don't want diabetes to ruin a perfectly lovely evening. I can fix this."
Now, you say to the waiter: "Please come back in a minute for our order." (Great, eh? Control the situation!)
You say to your family: "When you try to control my life, even when you are well meaning and correct, I resent it and often deliberately try to do the opposite."
They feel: Sort of relieved; no fight and no cake, yet.
They say: "You're right. We'd probably react the same way. How can we take care of our concern *and* your feelings?"
You feel: Respected, pleased.
You say: "I'm glad we're talking about this. I actually like you to say something for your sake and mine. Please just *ask* me before you *tell* me what to do. You could say, "I'd like to share a thought that you might find helpful—or possibly annoying." (You all laugh).
You all smile: The cake might not even be necessary; good cheer is quite filling.

It may sound rehearsed, but it must be in the beginning, if you are going to change old thinking and communication patterns. Your goals can be to have strong self-esteem, good relationships, and good diabetes control. Poor self-esteem or disturbed family relationships can be a complication of diabetes. You can treat these with the serum of self-knowledge, self-respect, hardiness, respect for others, and skillful interactions.

1. **Self-knowledge:** Know what you are feeling. Anger? Disappointment? Annoyance? Burnout? Resentment?
2. **Self-respect:** Accept your need for these feelings as part of the disease process.
3. **Hardiness:** Feel capable of controlling challenges, feelings, and tasks.
4. **Respect:** Acknowledge the needs and feelings of your friends, family, and others.
5. **Skillful interactions:** Find your comfort level and pass it on to family, friends, co-workers, and medical team.
6. An **interaction plan** for your family discussions should include
    - *what* needs to be said
    - *how* to say it and
    - *when* to say it.

Creating healthy communications around diabetes gives all of you an opportunity for positive growth. Dealing with diabetes can help you instill the values that any family wants to have—unconditional love, mutual respect, warm communication, and mutual growth through positive, accurate feedback.

Good Mourning: Grieving and Putting You Back Together

Mourning is a necessary place to start, even though it usually comes at the end of something. For that matter, it is sometimes necessary to go back and do it again. Grieving—which is personal and different for each individual—can have a common thread of stages that must be completed by you and your family.

Any major loss brings about a mourning process, a sequence of emotional and physical stages. Mourning is part of having diabetes because

1. It explains the natural feelings that may follow the diagnosis of diabetes for you and your family.
2. It suggests there is an end; you will heal and move on from the intensity of your feelings.

The diagnosis of diabetes always comes as a blow. It has an impact on your emotions, your body, your daily life, and your future. The grief process leads the way to a positive attitude and acceptance of the daily and future challenges of diabetes. You are told that diet, exercise, and medication are the three parts of the diabetes treatment package. A fourth—and perhaps most powerful part—is recognition and treatment of your emotions.

DIABETES IS A MAJOR LIFE CHANGE

The mourning process is as necessary in diabetes as it is in any major life change. My father died when my sisters and I were 3, 5, and 7 years old. I think the three of us and my mom—together or separately—never really completed mourning the death of my father. This unexpressed grief has preoccupied us our whole lives. We girls were not allowed to talk about him. We had to let him go on our own and figure out, without talking about it, what it meant to us individually and as a family.

I decided to be proud of being different—what a wonderful bunch we were without a father. I never spent any time being jealous, competitive, angry, or sad. I had only one way to deal with his loss—to be fiercely positive. It was a very, very narrow path. As an adult, I've found that being positive is required if you want to be productive, but I had feelings left over. As I finished my own grieving process through psychotherapy, I could be more comfortable with my own difficult emotions. Eventually, I wasn't as afraid of my own or anyone else's. As Elie Wiesel said, "A tale of despair is a tale against despair."

It could have been worse. My attempts to adapt could have been less socially acceptable. I could have picked bitterness or despair as my perspective. Some of you may recognize a similar one-track mind in yourselves. For example, you may recognize that you have stayed angry or frightened or helpless ever since the diagnosis of diabetes. Perhaps, you are lodged deeply in denial. Denial is good for a while. It keeps you feeling safe. It keeps you from feeling all the other feelings that you don't want. However, when you miss a doctor's appointment because you don't want to face his judgment or your anger or fears, your denial is no longer healthy. You are beginning to get into trouble. Once you have good self-care habits in place, a level of "healthy denial" keeps the anxiety away. If you do not fulfill your need to complete the grieving process, you risk being continually depressed, anxious, nonadherent, or in denial. Others may go on to develop diabetes-related eating disorders.

WHAT IS GRIEVING?

Exactly what is the grieving process? Dr. Elisabeth Kubler-Ross is a psychiatrist who recognized a pattern to grief and defined the stages that individuals and their families naturally move through. She identified a beginning stage of denial, (numbness and isolation); a midstage marked by periods of anger, bargaining, and depression (beginning the awareness of what it all means); and finally, a stage of acceptance of one's feelings and the situation. In diabetes, the end stage of grief is not being overcome by the loss but having a renewed determination to live a full life.

Again, these stages are defined by feelings, thoughts, and behaviors. A man who is beginning to develop a complication and is in the denial stage might find himself working extra hours and avoiding diabetes care. A child in depression might be cranky and irritable. An adolescent in anger might be pumping out critical or put-down remarks. Sometimes it is a relief of great tension when a family can identify those difficult behaviors as part of a grief reaction. Knowing there will be a natural end to negative or obnoxious behavior, or that the parents or spouse can help end it after everyone takes some time, is very comforting.

On occasion in family therapy, I suggest the family pick a date that marks the end of the amnesty period given to a grieving child or adult who has been particularly annoying to the family. "You must allow Tim, age 10, (or Mr. Smith, age 55,) to be a brat for 6 more weeks. He must not lessen the frequency of his outbursts until then. Please make sure he has the right encouragement to go full steam ahead. After January 15, he will be expected to be upsetting for only a normal amount of time." With this, the family gets a different perspective, realizing that the problems they're having are normal. They can reasonably expect that things will settle down.

CRISIS

Whereas the grief process in diabetes will look different for every family, the basic underlying themes will be the same. The unique details are the preexisting strengths and weaknesses in the family—communication patterns, support, previous coping with loss and change, religious or spiritual connection, and, of course, individual personalities. When the initial diagnosis of diabetes is made, it's a good time for the health care team and the family to take a look at their past and present coping skills and styles. The results of this evaluation might suggest the need for professional help during the initial crisis. In diabetes, this is especially crucial because coping will require, for the rest of your life, healthy ways of facing and acting on the challenges in your life.

GRIEF AND LIFE-STAGES

The mourning process usually begins at the time of diagnosis, with or without you being conscious of it. It can reoccur at different points of normal development over your lifetime when the impact of diabetes takes on new meanings for you.

Mourning can also occur when there's any hint of complications of diabetes. Complications often feel like a new diagnosis, not just an outgrowth of diabetes.

Sharon, at 27, has had type 1 diabetes for 20 years. When she came in for a routine visit, her blood pressure was high. She became hysterical. The medical resident examining her came out of the room, panicked, looking for help with this patient who had an emotional problem. After an intensive exchange of information and perspectives, he began to understand the emotional problem was his, too. He was frightened by her fear, sadness, anger, and guilt. Those feelings are all normal responses for a person who is afraid that complications—in this case, high blood pressure—are beginning. Sharon feared that she would now get all the other possible complications. I helped the resident realize that his anxiety was also normal and gave him some direction to help him explore her feelings with her. He went back in to listen to Sharon. He did a really nice job for himself and her by treating both their reactions as normal. He felt powerful because he did not run from her fear. He helped her become more powerful by enabling her to face and share her fears. Together they were able to figure out a way to control her diabetes emotionally and medically. A primary ingredient of the plan they worked out was to include her family as part of the support team.

Sharon has continued to keep her blood pressure normal and has stayed healthy since that time, 10 years ago.

HOW IT FEELS

Grieving is a process that brings up many uncomfortable feelings. These are normal and healthy. There can be a rush, in the beginning or at points along the way, of very intense and extreme emotions that come cycling through with no particular order or warning. These can bring on a feeling of being out of control. It probably makes some people worry that they are going crazy, losing their memory or concentration, or now have a new negative hostile personality, in addition to diabetes!

They can be embarrassed by their anger at the doctors and their families or frustrated by their inevitable self-pity. They may feel that they are so different that no one else has a clue to how badly they feel or what it is like. This emotional pain often causes them to withdraw from others. This isolation makes others begin withdrawing too, not knowing the right thing to say.

You cannot make it your goal not to have these feelings. You can make it your goal not to let these feelings take over your life. Sometimes the grieving process can begin again perhaps a year after diagnosis, on the anniversary, when the realization hits that diabetes is not going away. You will move beyond these feelings. My patients show me this time after time.

THE FAMILY'S GRIEF

When you are diagnosed with diabetes, everyone in the family goes through loss and change. Their central concern, usually, is to love and care for you. Although they shouldn't, spouses, siblings, or children often feel selfish taking time to honor their own natural but uncomfortable feelings. When the numbness thaws out, family members can find themselves feeling resentful of the time and money required by diabetes management. They, too, can ask "why me?" They can be angry that you seem less available, more moody. They can be jealous that others are free from these pressures. They may feel guilty in trying to trace the cause or in not having seen it coming. They can certainly be feeling guilty that they are even having these feelings; after all, it's not nice to be angry at you who has enough problems to bear.

Donald, 11 years old and the loving big brother of Tony, age 5, was off at summer camp, feeling the pleasures of freedom from his family, occasional pangs of homesickness, and a sense of well-being from being an adored child. He anticipated homecoming to be the same every year. His parents and brother would surround and hug him. Then they'd go to dinner. He would tell stories about camp and his friends and catch up on the news at home. No matter how full they were, they'd top it off with ice cream.

As the bus drove into the terminal, he looked for the happy faces of his family. Donald's heart sank when he saw only his father. He was incredibly disappointed. When his father hugged him and began to cry, he knew that something was very wrong. His brother was in the hospital, with diabetes, and his mother was at Tony's side. Donald was sad and worried for his little brother. He was also angry that he had lost his special night.

As time went on, it seemed there were no more lighthearted moments. It was not Donald's imagination that Tony got all the attention. Mealtime was extremely annoying. Trips for ice cream were out of the question. It was hard not to feel resentment. It was also hard for Donald not to feel ashamed that he was bitter when Tony was obviously suffering much more than he was.

In the middle of a grief process, it looks like people are stuck in the middle of misery, too. Time and time again, I see individuals and their families cross this river and get to the other side. People often recall 6 months, 1 year, 2 years later how overwhelmed they were. In Donald's case, for a long time, he would lament over the night that his whole life changed. With time, both Tony and Donald turned their attention back to the good old "other" things in their lives—grades, friends, sports, humor. Diabetes was there. So were many other things.

Dr. Maria Kovacs, a psychologist at the University of Pittsburgh, has shown through research that by the end of the first year of diagnosis, her sample of families was back to being stable. Her work shows that there is increased distress in the beginning and supports the idea of stages in the grieving process. You and your family will move on.

A distinctly different father was Mr. Samuels, the father of a 14-year-old girl with diabetes. The family was referred to me by the physician, who had problems with the dominating, aggressive, "difficult" father. After berating me about the short fuse, judgments, and impatience of the doctor, Mr. Samuels insightfully said to me, "Doesn't the doctor know this is difficult and horrible for me? The doctor should treat me with kid gloves even when I'm rude and impatient with him." Mr. Samuels understood what was happening to him but couldn't control it at the time and desperately needed to be helped and cared for, in spite of himself.

Families and providers must be alert to the grief process so it doesn't get in the way of relationships or diabetes-care outcomes.

GRIEVING AND TYPE 2 DIABETES

There is a profound impact on adults who are diagnosed with type 2 diabetes and their families. Often the diagnosis—usually occurring after age 40—can trigger a midlife crisis. Aging is never easy. Most people go through a mourning process about growing older. Getting a chronic illness on top of having to adjust to getting older can intensify feelings of despair, fear, vulnerability, bitterness, or panic.

When you are diagnosed with diabetes, there is so much to learn, to do, to worry about. Your friends, going through their own midlife challenges, are planning week-long bike trips to test their bodies' strength. Your plans are about meals, medication, low blood sugar, and avoiding future complications. Sure, you're hearing a lot about exercise, but it seems like exercise is medicine, not fun. The money they spend on their pleasure trip looks like a better buy than the deductible for medical insurance and the cost of medical supplies for you. Jealousy and anger are lodged in your throat. You feel ashamed of being resentful of those dear friends who don't have health problems. Your feelings are maddeningly complex. The information you need to absorb to take care of your diabetes is even more so. You have to sort through feelings while trying to be poker-faced about the tasks of management. It's obvious that the only way to win with diabetes is to take care of it. It's not as obvious how to take charge of it.

If you are not mired in depression or anger, you are more able to meet the demands of managing diabetes. You feel happy when you are doing what you can to take care of yourself. In turn, the normal blood sugar levels that result create a biologically based good mood. The right amount of nutritious food, followed by the right amount of medication and exercise ensures that your brain is well fed and content. When your diabetes is under control, you feel better emotionally and physically. You feel in charge.

Tom was 48 years old, and his diabetes was discovered during a routine physical. Well, his wife made him go to the doctor because he had seemed tired, depressed, listless, and—her real complaint—he had no interest in sex. They had both attributed this to some kind of midlife thing. They figured that despite job promotions, financial stability, and success with their children and friendships, he must have somehow been overcome by getting older. In fact, his tiredness, fatigue, diminished sex drive, and temporary impotence were the result of very high blood glucose from his undiagnosed and untreated diabetes. It was not a midlife crisis after all. Their expectations about how they were supposed to feel about aging had masked an illness.

With the diagnosis of diabetes and its treatment—diet and exercise—part of his daily routine, Tom felt better. He had energy, optimism, and libido. There was a bounce in his step. This lasted for a long time. Then, one day, Tom came in to talk to me. Although he was feeling well enough, he started also feeling anxious and angry about having diabetes for the rest of his life. Tom was mourning over his diagnosis of diabetes. The diagnosis had also pushed him into thinking about aging. He was now in a funk about both. He was angry that he felt imprisoned by diabetes and because he was getting older. He needed to get over feeling sorry for himself before he let it keep him from taking care of himself.

Tom began to understand himself better after venting his anguish. He had already seen that his efforts in diabetes did make a difference in how he felt and in his blood glucose levels.

Actually, diabetes and a midlife crisis require the same coping skills. This means learning to let go of unrealistic expectations. It means giving up the need to control everything. For both conditions, you must make the mental shift to put yourself at the top of your list of priorities. Applied to diabetes, this means eating lunches and snacks on time rather than answering three more phone calls at work. You'll have to learn to let others assist you when you need it, without feeling put down or incapable. With diabetes, this means calling the doctor or health care team for help. The point is to find pleasure in what you can control in your life—the efforts you make, your communication with others. You need to realize that each—life and diabetes—is a process, and you'll have many experiences along the way. Your goal with aging and diabetes is to accept the passage of youth but not the passage of vigor or curiosity. Baby boomers will help in changing the usual expectations of what people can do at 50, 60, 70, and 80 years of age, insisting on continued challenges and vitality of life until far beyond what used to be middle age. These are the "new passages" of life, a notion we can thank Dr. Levinson and Gail Sheehy for describing to us.

GETTING SUPPORT WITH THE NORMAL PROCESS OF GRIEVING

It is crucial to emphasize the word *normal* in beginning to understand mourning. People can be frightened by their feelings and want to ignore them or run from them. It is important to find comfort. The danger here is in seeking out destructive means—such as alcohol or drugs—to comfort yourself. The most effective way to come to terms with these frightening feelings involves support from other people. Emotional support is not a luxury. Dr. David Spiegel, an oncologist in California, found that his patients who joined a support group for patients with cancer survived twice as long as those who faced it alone.

Molly, 50 years old, was diagnosed at age 10 and remembers feeling that she could not find anyone to complain to in her emotionally chaotic family of two alcoholic parents and eight children. She never shared her anxieties or self-care needs with anyone. When she found a new support system in her marriage and new family, she slowly revealed her issues with diabetes and stopped concealing her fears. A diabetes support group became a new, loving family that helped her get in touch with her anger and anxiety.

She began to lessen her grip on the fierce independence that she had adopted as a child. She began to accept help with her diabetes and her anxiety and inhibitions. When she reached menopause, she was shocked. She had never thought she would live that long! She was also astounded by her resentment at having to face the ordinary adjustments to growing older. Molly had been used to facing only the extraordinary challenges of diabetes. She was not sure she liked being normal, too. In time, she worked these feelings out.

SUPPORTING YOURSELF

If you can accept that difficult and unpleasant emotions are normal, you can begin to move forward in the healing process. **Recognition** of your feelings is the first step, followed by **expression** of those feelings. This can take many forms:

- Talking them out (sharing with other people who have diabetes, family, friends)
- Writing in a journal
- Exercise
- Creating through the arts or music

Once you achieve awareness and self-expression, you can be less fearful about the third step: reaching out to others for **support.** My interpretation of Dr. Spiegel's research is that support should probably be required—written down on the physician's prescription pad!

There are many who are put off by the notion of accepting support. Support may be seen as intrusive, annoying, or undermining independence. Make no mistake, the responsibility for your diabetes is ultimately yours. Self-reliance and support are not at odds.

Through this process—recognition, expression, finding support—you can reach acceptance of your feelings and eventually of the disease itself. This puts an end to the grieving. After accepting your feelings, you can reach the fourth step, **letting go.** Diabetes is enough of a challenge. You don't need to let unfinished business—guilt, anxiety, fear—hang around.

ACUTE AND CHRONIC ADJUSTMENT

With a new diagnosis or crisis, the patient is number one. The world needs to and should revolve around you. It's easy to do that for 10 days. When the realization hits that diabetes does not go away, the amount of energy that can be given to you has to change. You all have to change from the acute grief response, requiring very intense involvement, to the chronic grief response, needing a long-term balanced approach.

> **HEALING PROCESS**
>
> - Recognition
> - Expression
> - Support
> - Letting go

Coping: There Are Better Ways

We cope by figuring out how to live with our thoughts, feelings, behaviors, and health. We cope by developing our own responses to the demands from the outside world. Each of us has a personal coping style that seems to come naturally. Sometimes this natural response gets us short-term relief but is not always helpful in the long run. For example, you are going through a time in your life when you fear having a low blood sugar level in front of other people. If the way you cope with this fear is to **avoid** it or **escape,** you will say to yourself: "I'll think about preventing low blood sugar tomorrow and just let it be high today." This response can bring on a feeling of immediate relief. It also can bring on some nagging guilt or worry about the physical effects of high blood sugar for the rest of the day (irritability, thirst, excessive urination) or for the future (complications of diabetes).

Escape behaviors such as eating, smoking, sex, drinking, and drugs can create more problems for you and have a negative effect on your diabetes. This chapter introduces you to more effective coping methods that you can apply to the way you think and the way you react. The styles and strategies are universal—anyone can use them.

Sometime in my middle thirties, I developed a slight fear of flying. I coped with this anxiety by drinking a quick glass of wine right before the flight. I would usually take an evening flight and my remedy for coping went unnoticed in that I would join my cohorts in the airport bar.

Then I had to take early morning flights with my colleagues. My cover was almost blown. Being inventive, I would bring a small plastic bottle filled with wine to the airport, rush into the ladies room, close the stall door, and drink. This seemed to work in the short run; I was able to fly easily. However, it added new anxiety and concern about how I was using alcohol.

We can get used to coping in ways that don't seem to cause harm on the surface. Being able to look honestly at what we do is crucial. No one knew my secret, so I was able to sneak it past my own conscience for a while, too.

I found myself telling a close friend about my experiences with anxiety over flying. I told it as a funny story, but I heard something I didn't like. The worst part was feeling ashamed of my feelings and having a secret way of coping.

Telling a story about ourselves is a process that digs up what is buried and puts it out on the table. Many people write journals to get to these feelings. It is **naming** (out loud or in the privacy of a journal or diary) what feels intolerable. For me, humor made it palatable. I was actually using several coping mechanisms—**humor, ventilating** (telling stories), and **social support.** These help you recognize your own feelings and begin to adjust how you are handling certain aspects of your life.

I have heard many similar stories from patients who often use food or alcohol to cover their feelings of anger, anxiety, or loneliness. They are always relieved to emerge from isolation and shame when they first tell their stories—**name** their feelings—to me or in a diabetes support or therapy group.

What actually made me stop my airport drinking was a plane ride as a chaperone for 20 kids with diabetes on their way to diabetes camp. Caring about others **distracted** me and actually kept my anxiety from surfacing. Helping the kids forced me to come up with **rational thoughts** about taking a plane.

COPING SKILLS

1. Naming
2. Humor
3. Ventilation or story telling
4. Social support
5. Distraction
6. Altruism
7. Rational thought
8. Positive self-talk
9. Visualization
10. Empowerment
11. Assertiveness
12. Relaxation

When I distracted myself by thinking of others, I no longer focused on my own situation. At the same time I had an opportunity to see myself as valuable because I could help others. (**altruism**) Dr. Herbert Benson, in his book *Timeless Healing*, calls this the "helper's high." Support groups are an excellent place for this. Listening to and helping other people can help us gain a new sense of ourselves, thus adding to our self-esteem. It also allows us to see our own problems differently, when we hear how differently others view the same things. Distraction can be achieved also with things or activities such as audio books, reading, art, or music. Losing yourself in the act of creating—a painting, a clean floor, a carpentry project, a beautiful meal—is probably the best distraction of all, because it focuses and relaxes you.

Another coping strategy is to use **rational thoughts** to **challenge** the feelings that are natural but, if unchecked, can lead us astray. To apply **rational thought,** we must know what messages we give ourselves—not only what we feel but exactly what we say silently to ourselves. This has been referred to as our "internal dialogue" (Albert Ellis) or **self-talk.** Once we identify what we think, we can challenge these thoughts and change them.

There is nothing wrong with having troublesome thoughts at times. We all do. The skill is to recognize the *faulty thinking patterns*. Faulty ways of thinking are actually bad habits that can be relearned, once they are found. Thinking is powerful. It can send us in any direction, positively or negatively. If we challenge our irrational thinking, we can promote new behaviors that are healthy. Negative thoughts or attitudes can be grouped into categories. In the "Faulty Thinking Patterns" box are examples that you may recognize.

HOW TO CHALLENGE

To be able to challenge our thoughts and feelings, we must learn to detach ourselves. No, that would not be an out-of-body experience but an out-of-emotional turmoil experience. Once detached, **visualize** yourself as a compassionate coach who accepts your feelings and thoughts but can help you see yourself differently. (Yes, there are two of you.)

Faulty thoughts seem to be automatic. But you can learn to make the challenges to these thoughts automatic, too. The challenges can come as analysis or positive statements. Sometimes, only a slight effort can redirect faulty thinking, and sometimes deeper probing is necessary.

FAULTY THINKING PATTERNS

1. All or nothing: You look at feelings or situations in extremes only—black or white, good or bad. No room is made for all those shades of gray that exist in reality. Looking at the world with rigidity and harshness brings trouble. If you're not good, then you must be bad. Eating one cookie is the same as eating a whole bag. (**Challenge:** But not according to your blood sugars.)

Thought	Challenge
Person with diabetes: I ate a cookie. I finished the rest of the package. I'm a failure.	I did a nice job all day of taking care of myself. This is not a disaster. This is just a slip. I've only eaten two cookies. I don't have to eat the whole box. My blood sugar will be 180 instead of 400. Everybody slips. I'm not a failure. I'm just a person with a temporarily high blood sugar.
Expected outcome: Continue overeating and bad feelings.	**Expected outcome:** Good mood enables you to make a plan for getting blood sugar down.

Thought	Challenge
Family member: I yelled at my child. I'm a terrible, selfish parent.	I yelled because I was angry. I'm human. I can be a great member of this family *and* lose control. She can be a great kid, have diabetes, and sometimes deserve to be yelled at. I'm okay.
Expected outcome: Feeling so badly, continues to yell.	**Expected outcome:** Feeling better, feels loving and generous to self and child.

continued

2. Never or always thinking: This thinking comes from wanting perfection. Shoulds and musts provide little chance of being successful. It's a setup for feelings of failure.

Thought	Challenge
Person with diabetes: I should *never* be depressed. It makes me overeat.	I'm human. Sometimes I will be depressed. I'll get over it. I always do. I'll help my depressions in ways other than eating.
Expected outcome: Feeling like a failure, overeats to feel better.	**Expected outcome:** Allowing for imperfection, moves on to something better.

Thought	Challenge
Family member: I must never be depressed. It's not fair to my husband who has enough with his diabetes.	For my own sake, I will try to be as happy as I can. I know my good mood pleases him, too. If I am upset, he is distracted from his problems and can be loving to me.
Expected outcome: Can't live up to perfection, gets more guilty, depressed.	**Expected outcome:** Feels relieved, less burdened by spouse's response, has more energy.

3. Selected negativity: You pay attention only to the negative details. You focus on the problem in a situation. (dark versus rose-colored glasses.) This leaves you with a negatively biased and therefore inaccurate view of your experiences. You must focus on the positive aspects of yourself, your life, and the people in it.

Thought	Challenge
Person with diabetes: Nobody will ever love me because I have diabetes.	First, do *I* love me since I have diabetes? It's just a part of me. Not my favorite part. I'm not in a relationship now. I've always been able to find love. I will again. I'm really a great person—who has diabetes.
Expected outcome: Feels bad, leading you to isolation from others. You end up alone because of your attitude, not diabetes.	**Expected outcome:** Feels better, goes to social functions to meet and interact with other people.

Thought	Challenge
Family member: No matter how much I try to help her, she yells and doesn't appreciate me.	I like how much I help my wife with her diabetes. When she is in a bad mood, she sometimes yells at me, and at everyone else. Her anger doesn't mean she doesn't appreciate me. Come to think of it, I am bossy sometimes.
Expected outcome: Feels sorry for self and withdraws or becomes argumentative.	**Expected outcome:** Relaxed by thinking, doesn't overreact to wife's anger.

continued

4. Emotional focus: This thinking fuels our false belief that how we feel is the way things are.

Thought	Challenge
Person with diabetes: I'm depressed. I'm going to get diabetes complications.	So, I'm depressed. Period. I'm in good health. Feeling bad does not cause complications. Bad feelings pass. I can be frightened, pessimistic. Those are feelings. They are not my reality. I take care of myself. I can continue my good health.
Expected outcome: Depressed, doesn't take care of self.	**Expected outcome:** With focus on positive perspective—after ventilation of bad or worried feeling—calls for doctor's appointment for motivation and reassurance.

Thought	Challenge
Family member: I feel terrible. I ate candy in front of my sister with diabetes. I'm a very bad person.	I am not perfect about being nice to my sister all the time. I have feelings and needs, too. They are different from her needs. I am a normal, good, kid.
Expected outcome: Feels badly, resents sister more.	**Expected outcome:** Feels better about self and sister.

POWER IN THINKING AND ACTION

If you are used to dealing with doctors with a dependent, passive, fix-my-illness approach, empowerment brings an independent, active, team-oriented (with you in the center) approach.

Robert, 10 years old, was a delightful, intelligent, well-adjusted child. With the diagnosis of diabetes, he seemed to adapt well, never breaking stride with his good grades. Some months after his diagnosis, his mother called to say that his grades had fallen, and he did not seem interested in inviting any of his friends to come over after school anymore. As their concern increased, they finally brought Robert in for a visit. He revealed that he had had a devastating experience. In class one day, a rumor had begun that Robert's diabetes was contagious. Shocked and hurt, he was unable to answer. The kids assumed that the rumor was true and were afraid to be close to him. He was too overwhelmed and embarrassed to tell anyone. He did not want his parents to know because they had been upset enough about the diabetes. He felt he had caused enough turmoil already.

Robert's parents were tremendously relieved to hear his story. They laughed and cried and hugged him. Robert, who was so sure that they would be disappointed in him, was immensely relieved, too. Because they had been telling him all along that they were so proud of how strong he was and how he never complained, he felt he could not let them down now. He had decided to handle it all by himself. This was such a nice turning point for the whole family. The family's way of coping was to be positive and protective of each other and only share the good things. It was a relief to all of them to be more open about the hard parts, too.

Robert began to understand that he would probably have been afraid of another child's diabetes. What had seemed like rejection could now be seen as fear and not enough knowledge. He decided to give a talk to the class, with another older child in the school who was very well liked and had diabetes, too. The closing line, which he delivered with a twinkle in his eye, was: "Just remember, diabetes is catching only if I don't like you!" Everyone laughed. After identifying his feelings and getting support, he was able to think differently about his experience. He also could teach others how to think differently about his diabetes. Diabetes was bringing him more, not less, power.

In a support group for parents of newly diagnosed children, the issue had come up that one of their children, Amy, age 8, had not been invited to a birthday party by one of her good friends. The mother, Mrs. S, and the group were angry. Mrs. S felt rejected, hurt, and inferior. We could feel her self-esteem falling as she told us the story. The group consensus was that Amy should drop the friend because she was obviously not a good friend.

These things would probably happen again. Each time it would be easy, but not healthy, to take the path of bitterness and resentment. A more difficult response, but one that is ultimately more satisfying, would be to try doing something. We worked out an assignment: Mrs. S would call the other mom.

The friend's mother was apologetic. She said that she had not wanted to put Amy into the terrible position of not being able to eat birthday cake, ice cream, and candy. Ashamed of being selfish, the mother admitted that she was afraid Amy might get sick and that she might not be able to help her. Mrs. S swallowed hard. Those were honest admissions, but they still made her angry. Mrs. S then said, after many deep breaths, "I'm glad you told me. I don't really feel good about what you've said, but I do appreciate your being honest with me. I'd like Amy to come to the party. She'll have fun with her friends. She can eat the cake, with a little planning ahead about extra insulin or more play time. Sounds like you need another chaperone, anyway. Why don't I come and give you a hand with the kids?"

It was tough emotionally, but Mrs. S turned the situation around. She set the tone that no one needed to be afraid of Amy. They could just enjoy her company and friendship. She realized what a tremendous amount of **assertiveness** she was going to need and that eventually Amy would need the same skills that Robert did in the previous story. Mrs. S was still angry, but the power of taking action rather than feeling like the victim was enough to dissipate the fury she had originally felt. She saw this as an excellent example of how **social support** enabled her to let out her rage in an environment of acceptance.

Lena was diagnosed with type 1 diabetes as a young woman. She spent many years trying to cope with her internal reactions (anger, guilt, frustration, and inadequacy) to her husband's and her mother's comments about what she ate and how she lived. When she felt put down by their comments on her eating, she had a plan. In fact, she had her plan written down on an index card:

1. *Think about what you are feeling.*
2. *Think of some other way besides eating to handle the feeling.*
3. *Make yourself feel better. Find comfort.* ***(distraction)***
   a. *Get a skim milk cappuccino*
   b. *Suck your thumb, literally. (In private) Pouting can be good for the soul.*
   c. *Call a friend and leave an unbelievably long message on her machine if she is not home.*
   d. *Rent a movie.*
   e. *Take a walk. If necessary, take an even longer walk.* ***(relaxation)***
4. *Give effective feedback to unintentionally injuring parties.*

COMMUNICATION

With an empowered attitude and good coping skills, you can move from positive self-talk to having effective communication with the people in your life.

> Bob is a patient with type 2 diabetes, and this is a conversation he had with his wife.
>
> **Bob's wife:** How much longer are you going to go around feeling sorry for yourself and hurting everyone's feelings with your sarcasm and bitterness?
> **Bob:** Probably about 3 more months, but only if you stop judging me for my anger. You'd be angry, too. And even if you wouldn't be, I am. That's me.
> **Bob's wife:** You're right. I'm impatient because I feel so inadequate that I can't help you. I suppose it seems like I'm judging you, but I think I'm really judging myself. And I miss my fun partner.

Although it often appears that the issues in type 2 diabetes are conflicts over food or body image, they may actually be the issues in all marriages—control and self-control. Both the person with diabetes and the person without it may feel like a victim. Because food is part of our daily lives, the feelings and interactions surrounding eating need to encourage emotional well-being and good diabetes control.

Joe, age 58, with type 2 diabetes for 6 years, has a very close and loving relationship with his younger sister Jane, age 50. They were, however, locked in an emotional cold war regarding his diabetes. He resented the comments she made without permission on the personal aspects of his life. He felt more vulnerable about diabetes in public because he was talked about and criticized in the family circle. His sister felt rejected and furious that he seemed to care so little about himself and his health and made those around him feel so helpless.

INEFFECTIVE COPING METHODS

- Denial
- Avoidance
- Escape (for example, excessive eating or drinking)
- Acting out (for example, daring behavior or anger)

Their ways of coping with the stresses they felt changed over time, but in the beginning, Joe deliberately ate more in front of the family, daring them to judge him. Defying them gave him a strange sense of power. (aggression, not **empowerment**) He expressed his resentment and hostility through his behavior. Analyzing this later, he determined that he had made his family the scapegoat to avoid feeling his fury at having diabetes and the restrictions and fears that came with it. His sister had reacted to his overeating with alternating bouts of rage and coldness. On reflection, she saw that it was easier for her to be angry and controlling towards him, than to feel sadness and fear about what he had to go through.

The ways they each seemed to cope, whether denial, avoidance of the real feelings and issues, or acting out behaviors (his daredevil eating and her excessive anger), all interfered with their relationship and with his health. The communication that grew between them, after several therapeutic breakthroughs, gradually broke down the barriers.

ASSERTIVE COMMUNICATION SKILLS

1. Assertion: direct, honest, concise statements of feeling, need, or thought
2. Listening
   a. Repetition: repeat what you think you heard using "I" statements, staying on target, avoiding interruptions
   b. Clarification: try to find out if what you think you heard was correct
3. Assertive empathy: honest compassion stated clearly at the beginning of your response
4. Assertive request: simply clarify what you need
5. Positive assertion: highlight the positive: (part of positive reframing)
6. Agreement: nondefensive posture

Assertions are concise, straightforward comments that tell the feeling or idea without demeaning anyone. Good communication comes from assertions followed by good listening, empathy, and a nondefensive attitude. The first rule of good communication is to respect each other's right to speak openly and to take turns. You also need to accept and forgive strong emotions from each other at times.

> **Joe:** This is none of your business. I'll do what I want. You can't control me.
> **Jane:** My interest and my questions feel controlling? **(listening)**
> **Joe:** They sure do. You, the doctors, my wife...I don't have a life. **(agreement)**
> **Jane:** That sounds awful for you. **(assertive empathy)**
> **Joe:** Thanks. It is. I feel like my privacy is gone, like everyone is free to intrude on me the first moment I do something wrong. I've always eaten terribly, and with all the anxiety about this illness, I can't seem to start changing my relationship with food now.
> **Jane:** I'm so glad you're telling me this. **(positive assertion)** I don't want you to do this alone. **(assertion)** Can we figure out some way that I can be your friend and not a critic? **(assertive request)**
> **Joe:** Maybe, but don't get carried away.
> **Jane:** Well, thank you for talking to me about this. Now I will be happier being able to communicate with you, and I have a feeling that will make life better for you too. **(positive assertion)**

COPING HELPS WITH THOSE FEELINGS

Again, you start by **recognizing** your own feelings, and then those of others. When you identify feelings, you can step away from their power over you. You don't have to act on them. Remember the power of the insert? This next step allows you to **desensitize** yourself—step back and take the sting out of your feelings. Jane did this when she was able to step back and hear her brother, knowing that the time to express her feelings would come. Another part of coping is to **anticipate** life's situations. Then you can **prepare** so you are not caught off guard and can handle events or people who might upset you. After all, we find out what the weather will be to decide what shoes to wear or whether we will carry an umbrella. In a similar way, we can prepare for everything from criticism from family members to the tempting foods at parties.

JOE'S THOUGHTS

Recognize: I really get anxious and feel like overeating whenever I go to a party with family or friends who know about my diabetes.
Desensitize: Relax. Anybody would be nervous. I'm no different. I can feel that way but I don't have to act that way. **(rational thoughts)**
Anticipate: I really have to figure out a new way to react when Jane stares at my plate. I don't want to overeat, and I don't want to be angry with her.
Prepare: I know what I can say if she bugs me. My humor always softens her. I'll say, "I'm so happy to *see* you. I'm not as happy to *hear* you." Then I will use **visualization,** picturing in my mind how good I will feel after this kind of improved interaction.

JANE'S THOUGHTS

Recognize: I'm starting to be nervous about going for dinner with Joe. By the time I work myself up, I'll be angry, too.
Desensitize: Relax. Anybody would be nervous. When you love someone and you see them hurting themselves, you get impatient with them. **(rational thoughts)**
Anticipate: I'm going to be relaxed and loving tonight and not look for a fight to get him to change or help me get rid of my frustration.
Prepare: I'm ready for this. I will sit *next* to Joe so I don't have to watch what he does. I'll grab his arm with warmth. He's a sucker for my sisterly love. And now I

will think about how nice this will feel. **(visualization)** Again we see that you and your family members can be both empathetic and hurting. There are no bad guys here. Families have a tremendous capacity to help each other.

You will use these coping skills everyday, and they will become as natural as breathing. Well, they'll be as natural as following a meal plan or taking insulin has become. These skills can prevent the overload that diabetes can bring and can be applied to all stresses in your life.

It is helpful for newly diagnosed people and their families to get counseling for good mental health and to create a foundation to meet the challenges ahead. This is as important as taking care of yourself physically. Our culture has begun to ease the old stigmas about psychotherapy, but people can resist it for many reasons. They may feel that it is a weakness to need help or that something is terribly wrong. As a colleague of mine and I wrote in *Diabetes Forecast* many years ago, "You don't have to be crazy to see a therapist, but sometimes you have to be crazy not to." Ideally, the mental health therapist is already or will become a part of the health care team. To find the right counselor, ask for recommendations for someone who has experience with either diabetes or chronic illness. Make sure you are comfortable with the therapist. You can call several agencies either locally or nationally for referrals in your area.

What's So Special about Support?

Support is central to taking care of diabetes. This chapter is about the role that support can, and hopefully does, play in your life. Simply:

1. Give it.
2. Get it.
3. Learn to recognize it.
4. Give just enough of it.
5. Give it unconditionally. (without necessarily getting anything in return)
6. Give some of it to yourself.

KINDS OF SUPPORT

People with diabetes can use family support, support groups, or therapy to develop a strong, positive identity. I have seen support give welcome relief, a chance for ventilating difficult emotions, new perspectives, optimism, a positive spin on an incredibly difficult experience, and even improvement in diabetes management.

Support can take many forms. It can be informational (facts and techniques), emotional or spiritual (dealing with inner feelings and values), or tangible (concrete tasks or services).

In a support group meeting, Susan, 21, finds out how to manage her diabetes if she decides to have a drink. ***(informational)*** *She also is confronted with the emotional aspects of where and when she might want to drink. Does she fear being different? Does she have to prove herself to everybody else? Does she not drink in front of others, fearing they will comment on her behavior? Does she drink privately or in binges?* ***(emotional)*** *The group would then help her come up with a self-awareness exercise, recording her feelings and behaviors during the week and reporting back to the group at the next session.* ***(tangible)***

In the same group, Don, age 60, is shocked and upset that he must go for some laser surgery on his eyes. The group listens to his fears, anger, and guilt and asks him questions that encourage him to expand on his feelings. ***(emotional)*** *When he is able, he takes information from members of the group that can quiet his fears, for example, that laser treatment can stabilize retinopathy and prevent further damage to his eyes.* ***(informational)*** *A group member offers to take Don to his appointment.* ***(tangible)***

At the next few meetings, other group members discuss their anxiety at being so close to someone who is experiencing diabetes complications. In fact, this experience makes them face their worst fears. In comforting one another, they realize that they can handle whatever might happen to them—especially if they are not alone. The group members begin to talk about monitoring their own blood glucose more closely. This does not come exclusively from fear. Improving their *efforts* at normalizing blood glucose levels—the part they can control—has always been a main focus of the group. These efforts increase their chances of living long and healthy lives. Their efforts to confront their fears and strive to do their personal best boost self-esteem, and this helps them with diabetes management, too.

MEN AND WOMEN

The kind of support you like depends on your personality, your cultural background, and your sex. There is a lot of useful information about the differences between men and women (gender differences) and the way each goes about expressing a need for and giving support. Deborah Tannen *(You Just Don't Understand)* and John Gray *(Men Are From Mars, Women Are From Venus)* both emphasize the need to understand rather than judge our different styles of relating to each other.

Men and women both need to know the comfort to be gained in giving and getting support. Often men are taught that receiving support means they are weak. This is a problem for men who have diabetes. If the cultural and social influences are spelled out, then a man can understand his attitudes and feel more open to changing them to help his diabetes. You can more effectively take care of diabetes when you don't have to do it alone, in a vacuum.

For every person, just having someone listen to your feelings is often enough.

Mary complains to her husband John that she was humiliated when she had a reaction during her workout at the gym and never wants to return there. John really wants to help her. He says, "Who cares what others think?" He jumps to trying to help her problem-solve what she can do to avoid low blood sugar levels at the gym (information she already has). John really loves Mary, and he wants to support her. He cannot understand why this makes her furious. She yells at him that he has no patience and is always lecturing. Now, despite his good intentions, they are in a fight. She is yelling, and he is cold and withdrawing because she has rejected his support. Mary, misinterpreting his support, wanted him to put his arms around her and just listen to her feelings.

When John tells Mary that he is upset with his mother-in-law because she criticizes him for not watching Mary's eating habits more closely, he can't stand that Mary has to ask so many questions and go on and on about it. To him, her comments and questions feel like nagging, which only adds to the problem. That is why John—who wants to talk to Mary—doesn't like to tell Mary about his other personal interactions and feelings. Ironically, Mary, too, is craving closeness with her husband. She would give anything to figure out how to open him up and help him feel better and help her take care of her diabetes.

It is important not to stay locked in being chronically unfriendly and misunderstood. Neither masculine nor feminine approach to feelings or problems is superior. They are just different. With the strengths of both points of view working together rather than against each other, situations can be resolved on a higher level. Two heads are better than one!

Unfortunately, people tend to get stuck in their differences. Nancy and Sam, the parents of 7-year-old Susan, who has diabetes, have worked this problem out for some of their situations. When Susan, after taking her insulin shots, refused to eat what her mom made for dinner, Nancy would go into the kitchen to prepare something else, saying the whole time that it was okay, don't worry, anything for my baby. Sam would become furious and critical of both of them. He wanted his daughter eating now—with no back talk—whatever his wife had already made. He had no patience for either his wife or daughter. He thought them incompetent and manipulative, respectively.

In his masculine view, order is based on a vertical hierarchy of power and structure. As the dad, he felt that the parent sets the rules. His wife's female orientation is horizontal, emphasizing closeness, relationship, and discussion time. When we look at this situation, it seems clear to the outsider that the child needs the benefit of both orientations. She needs the boundaries, the respect, and the clear expectations of her father as well as the patience, interest, and effort to please of her mother.

Refusing to eat is an important issue that needs prompt attention to avoid low blood glucose. If left unsolved, this situation can lead to chronic mealtime tension. Good problem solving requires the input of both parents. Each has something to offer to the solution. The emotional support, patience, and understanding that Nancy offers are vital to the child. These need, however, to be complemented by Sam's no-nonsense style. Throw in a little intellectual detective work (Is she already low? would that account for her negativity? Did she eat a candy bar or other food without telling anybody and know that she doesn't need to eat much more? Is she simply not hungry? Is this a new developmental power struggle?) Now we are on the way to making mealtimes work better for all of them.

Both Nancy and Sam were on the mark. They understood they were becoming opponents rather than partners who share the same goals. Sam supported Nancy by learning to listen to her frustration. She was able to support him by appreciating how clearly he could see the situation. The plan they developed was to have Sam hold Nancy's hand, making his support concrete for her and reminding her to stay strong. It also reminded him not to lose his temper, his former way of helping. (They thought this was corny and unrealistic at first.) Nancy would then ask her daughter why she didn't want to eat, would listen and try to understand her response, and then clearly state the choice that they would allow. In this case, they had decided that Susan must join them at the dinner table, because they wanted her company. If she didn't want to eat what was being served, she could choose to make her own cheese or peanut butter sandwich for her dinner one or two times a week. Any low blood glucose levels at dinnertime would be treated with glucose tablets so as not to ruin her appetite, or sweets would be worked into the meal plan, ahead of time, as part of dinner.

They could have solved this issue using any one of many satisfactory approaches. What felt good to Nancy and Sam was that they felt closer to each other and had a new respect for the value of each point of view. Sam stopped being irritated with his wife and daughter. He opened up about how he worried about his daughter. He felt responsible for her doing the right things without actually knowing what those things were. He began to learn more about diabetes, so he would have more patience and provide real help with the diabetes. The relationship between Sam and his daughter became closer. She received positive attention from him about her diabetes. Sam helped Nancy keep from burning out on their daughter's diabetes management. She did not have to go to excessive lengths to please her daughter. Being loving but firm—her new image of herself—pleased Nancy and her daughter just fine.

SUPPORTING TOO MUCH

Determining whether support is welcome and helpful is the other side of the story. There is support that strangles the receiver. Taking too much responsibility for another can leave that person feeling inadequate or angry.

For years, I ran family support groups and gave support, advice and even confrontation when necessary. I enjoyed getting along so well with the kids. The tide turned when I spent time at diabetes camp as a counselor. Many of them remarked on the change in me. In switching from my neutral supportive role to that of a parent substitute, I became more nagging, anxious, impatient, and controlling. The kids wanted me kicked out of the cabin. I had a new profound respect for how difficult it is to be a family member and still be respectful and respected.

One father had been well meaning but highly anxious and intrusive in his 18-year-old daughter's life. In the course of family therapy, she realized that she had stopped taking any interest in her diabetes because it seemed that her father cared enough for both of them. She did not tell anyone that she had diabetes because she assumed that everybody would respond as he did—nervous, nagging, and critical. She resented him because she thought that in his eyes, she was a burden, an unsuccessful diabetic, rather than a beloved daughter with diabetes. She just wanted to be loved and respected as a person, so no one else in her life was going to know about her diabetes. The father and the daughter had a lot of painful work to do. A balanced amount of caring and support from her father was what she needed so she could do the right things for her diabetes.

THE HEALTHY WAY TO RECEIVE SUPPORT

It is sometimes difficult to realize that true support happens only when we care about and love ourselves, first. When adults with diabetes are responsible for taking care of others, they often neglect their own needs and that includes diabetes.

Sam, age 46, works hard for his family and his boss. Sam runs out the door, forgetting to take his high blood pressure medication, skips lunch, grabs candy bars to keep from getting low, misses doctor appointments, and doesn't make time to reschedule the appointments. Starving by dinnertime, he eats huge portions while his wife looks on with criticism. After dinner, he falls asleep in his chair because of extremely high blood glucose levels, being too tired to exercise or engage in family time.

When asked, Sam knows that he just doesn't have time for himself. Supporting his family is more important than supporting himself. He puts all those hours in so they can be proud of him for his promotions and paychecks. At work, he cannot say no to requests from his co-workers. He would never let his boss down on the frequent last-minute rush jobs.

Sam does not have time for himself and therefore no time for diabetes. If a complication of diabetes occurs, Sam will be forced to make time for himself to try to pick up the pieces. For Sam to manage his diabetes and confront the pressures he is not dealing with, he would have to take some positive action to rearrange his priorities.

To support himself, he would have to realize he was a valued employee and could ask for fewer last-minute requests from his boss, order lunch to be delivered so he could eat at his desk, and say no to any appointments that interrupt his scheduled medical visits.

Anna, Sam's wife, became exhausted and frustrated by her unsuccessful involvement. She felt like a failure for not getting Sam to adhere to his diabetes regimen. She was hurt that he seemed to set limits only with her. Although she was right about what he needs to do, unfortunately, her original, sincere supportive stance had changed. Her love had been infiltrated by anger, resentment, and the desire to control. Her efforts to communicate consisted mainly of snide comments and rude stares. She had stopped making healthy meals. Anna began to gain weight and feel depressed. She felt unappreciated and angry at failing in her misguided goal—controlling her husband's health—and was missing out on any physical and emotional support from her husband.

On the other hand, Sam was feeling hurt that she no longer was supportive of him. He was right. Anna stopped her caretaking and her caring. She let his behavior become her focal point. She sacrificed her own health (weight gain) and mood in the process. In that way, they were alike. They both needed to realize that true support is about caring and loving themselves first. It is not about controlling another person or giving up one's own needs in the process. The kind of support he thought he was giving—making a living—was not the only support he or his family needed.

Anna and Sam both needed to dedicate more time and energy to themselves. To get and to give true support, they had to worry more about themselves than each other, discuss their feelings, figure out realistic expectations of each other, and begin—after this openness—to trust in each other's potential. Both of them needed to shift their focus from others to themselves.

Excessive support can lead to overinvolvement and an expectation that the other person must live in a certain way. These sometimes unvoiced and unmet expectations can lead to feelings of anger, disappointment, and criticism. The person who receives this kind of support can begin to feel incapable or dependent. These feelings can turn into depression or anger at oneself or toward the support giver.

Even if you don't have diabetes, it is necessary to nurture yourself and then to get others to nurture you, too. A relationship cannot survive if the people in it are not equal in importance and respect. You are just as important as your partner, even if your partner seems to be facing more challenges or problems than you.

TAKE CARE OF YOURSELF FIRST

I learned this when my husband had coronary bypass surgery. My sister Marcia had stubbornly, and wisely, insisted that she come along to support me as I supported my husband. Duh. If she had not been so strong in her beliefs about what I needed, I probably would have succeeded in resisting her. (It feels good to say no to an older sister.) So I was force-fed her support, thank goodness. I really did learn from her about taking better care of myself. I was lucky, too, that she was there.

While waiting for the surgery to be over, I had increasing pains in my chest. That is an embarrassing symptom to have while your husband is undergoing heart surgery. Talk about sympathy pains. Marcia insisted that I go to the doctor, once we knew the surgery was successfully completed.

The doctor told me that my pain was physically real, even though it was triggered by my stress. He gave me a medical explanation for the chest pain resulting from my anxious and shallow breathing pattern. I felt embarrassed being there. He teased me, chiding the psychologist for not respecting the power of the mind over the body.

HEALTHY SUPPORT

Built into healthy support is unconditional love, accepting people for who they are, regardless of their desire or their success in taking care of themselves. That means offering support in the form of challenge, advice, listening, or whatever, but only offering it—not insisting on it. Love cannot be based on people doing what pleases you. My other sister Mary Ellen reminds me to let other people live their own lives, and support them by pointing out their strengths and capabilities.

Loving unconditionally needs to go both ways. Both the nagging parent or spouse and the noncompliant child or adult need support. The person who appears nagging or controlling also needs honest feedback and unconditional love.

Sometimes we are disappointed in the patterns of support that we receive. People we count on get busy with aspects of their own lives. It is important to accept changes in the patterns of intimacy and commitment from our friends and relatives.

You may have unrealistic expectations of yourself and of others. You may be trying to control the situation too much. You can try to recognize and let go of anger and disappointment so that it doesn't color your relationships in the future. Negative feelings hurt you, not just your family and friends. You need to work at setting aside false pride and not let go of those who are important to you.

It is easy to get absorbed in self-pity or criticism, but if you are a "poor me" all the time, will your choices be limited? Changing this pattern requires forgiveness and learning to focus on giving love and compassion. Ask yourself the question: Do I want to be happy or correct? Most often, children choose to be happy. We can learn from them. They recuperate quickly from a fight and move on to play, holding no grudges.

Ben, at age 29, began to have a series of complications with his eyes, feet, and kidneys. We all felt sad and concerned for him. His family and the medical team had tried to be there for him during many years of his alcohol abuse and his diabetes. His sister came to me because of her anger and depression. She was furious at him for never listening to her and now found herself openly hostile to him. She could not bring herself to give him any support or the concrete help he needed. After she saw him, she would feel so guilty about the rage and rejection she felt for her little brother, who was obviously suffering the consequences of his diabetes and unhealthy behaviors.

After several sessions, she found some understanding about her guilt. She was upset with herself for two things. First, she had always carried guilt that it was her little brother and not her who had diabetes. Second, she felt she had not done enough to help him prevent complications, despite knowing that people can only influence, not control each other and that diabetes does not always respond to our efforts. In therapy, she could grieve about all this and was able to turn from anger and guilt to focus on the sadness and love she felt for her brother. She had to reach out to support him now. His own pain and loss allowed him to see and accept the support she had tried to offer him for years.

RX: SUPPORT

Support turns out to be good for your health. We take for granted that it feels good, but it actually is a form of medicine. It could be prescribed by your doctor. There is healing in the process of confiding, bonding, and developing attachments.

THE GOALS OF SUPPORT

Support is not about fixing; it is about being there. People and medical personnel often move away when they think they cannot do something to bring back your good health. Ironically, that is the time you may most need your family and health professionals. You need supportive people who do not fear the feelings of sadness or rage that are often part of the process of adjusting to change and loss.

GIVE SOMEONE ELSE SUPPORT

An interesting fact of life is that the time to support someone else is when you are most weary about the prospects of your own health. Giving support to others is a major positive distraction from being too self-absorbed. Focusing outward helps you balance your perspective. It also gives you a needed boost of energy and purpose. You can't help others without helping yourself.

Dean could not be moved from feeling angry at his diabetes and, as a result, was neglectful of it. He was estranged from his family and stubbornly refused to begin working things out with them. The holidays were coming. Dean had no plans. He wouldn't call friends to ask to be included. He was determined to hold on to his sorrow. We made a pact. Dean agreed to limit his sulking to 2:00 pm on Thanksgiving Day and then force himself to join a group that was feeding the homeless. Dean was shocked by the impact of the experience. In helping others, he could feel generous, grateful, and strong.

For the first time in a long time, he experienced liking himself. He realized his bitterness at being diagnosed had been the only thing he focused on. He also realized he must have alienated a lot of well-meaning people. Dean knew he wasn't cured yet of his resentment, but it felt good to remember that there were many times in his life that he had felt good about himself. I was crossing my fingers (part of my professional expertise) that he would continue helping out in that community group. His involvement was probably going to be as valuable as the therapy, antidepressants, and exercise prescription he was following.

Caring just enough allows you to feel good about the other person and allows the other person the freedom to accept or reject the help or caring. By giving you can learn to receive.

In an adult relationship, what we need from each other is "healthy detachment" (Melody Beattie, *Codependent No More)*. This means being loving and yet being two separate individuals. It suggests boundaries that say: "I have *my* place and you have yours." It requires that each person carry his load in being caring and responsive.

A FINE BALANCE

Reaching balanced support is hard to do. Why do all this? For you and the other person. So you won't go around being angry all the time. So s/he will feel competent and find no need to rebel against you or do everything you say to win your love. It promotes honesty. People can usually only tell the truth to people who don't overreact. Self-control and respect for each other encourages closeness, the kind of closeness that is not a burden for either one.

PERSON WITH DIABETES

Self-support: Your blood glucose reading is 300 mg/dl after what had seemed like a really excellent day. You say to yourself:

- **a.** No matter what I do, I can't help myself.
- **b.** I give up. Nothing works anyway.
- **c.** Something bad will probably happen to me anyway.
- **d.** Anybody would be frustrated. It is just a number. I can get it down by lunch. My usual blood sugars are in a very good range.

Answer evaluation: While **a, b,** and **c** can be satisfying, they are also defensive, self-deprecating, hostile, or downright aggressive. They are okay as private thoughts, to begin the process. **D** is more likely to help you feel positive.

continued

Giving support: Your wife has just yelled at you because all the cookies that were hidden in the pantry are gone.You say to her:

a. It looks like you have been eating them.
b. Picking on me because you had a bad day?
c. Your yelling is a turnoff.
d. I know you are yelling at me out of concern and worry. It sounds critical and mean when you yell. I will try to remember that it is coming from love and a desire to help. Thank you for that. I need to understand how difficult my diabetes is for you, too, sometimes.

Answer evaluation: Answer **a** would be good to say silently to yourself to make you laugh. Answers **b** and **c** have potential for you, making you feel you are not all that bad. Answer **d** takes work to get there but really helps you both.

Receiving support: At a dinner party, when the hostess serves dessert, she stops you from taking the cake and says out loud that you can't have that but she has baked you something special without sugar or fats. In a private conversation later, you say to her:

a. How dare you embarrass me like that!
b. Do you think you can control everyone like you do your husband?
c. Mind your own business.
d. Not many people have such a good friend who goes out of their way to understand diabetes as well as cook for it. Thank you. I feel close enough to tell you that I like to be private about my diabetes (no public discussions) and I like to make my own decisions about what to eat. Again, thanks for your efforts to help.

Answer evaluation: Answer **a** is honest, but **b** and **c** are downright hostile. Having the conversation later gives you the chance to cool off for answer **d.**

FAMILY MEMBER WITHOUT DIABETES

Self-support: You go into your 13-year-old daughter's room to make sure she is up for school and checking her blood glucose. She yells at you to get out, that you are always meddling in her life. You say to yourself:

- **a.** No matter what I do, I am no help to her or myself.
- **b.** I give up. What a failure I am as a parent.
- **c.** What an obnoxious, self-centered, unappreciative little brat.
- **d.** I will not take this personally. She seems to hate remembering that she has diabetes in the mornings. Actually, she was always grumpy in the morning even before she got diabetes. On the other hand, she is grouchy when she is a bit low. I am proud of myself for not getting upset at her or critical of myself. I will go back in with a blood glucose machine, some juice, and a smile.

Answer evaluation: Go directly to answer **d,** so you don't have to put yourself or your child down.

Giving support: Your husband complains that the result of your child's hemoglobin A_{1c} test is too high and that he was embarrassed and angry at you for not doing a good job with your son. You say to him:

- **a.** I am just not doing a good job at anything.
- **b.** Well, you should talk! You are distant, seldom here, and always critical of your son.
- **c.** I am sick of your put-downs.
- **d.** I can hear that you are just as upset as I am. I know it is tempting to blame me. I wish we could find someone to blame. Anything to give us some comfort. Let us be kind to each other in this disappointment. The hemoglobin is just a number that covers only a short period. We have to plan strategies together to help our son's control improve. Remember, the doctor said this is probably related to our son's going through puberty.

continued

Answer evaluation: Answer **c** is a conversation to have another time. Move on to honest, compassionate answer **d.**

Receiving support: Your husband's sister comes over to you at a party and exclaims that she can't believe you cannot take better care of your husband's diabetes. You say to her:

a. I know. I feel embarrassed that I can't stop him.

b. I don't see you helping **your** husband's drinking problem.

c. If you keep eating as much as you do, you will likely get it too. It is hereditary, you know.

d. Criticizing me is probably a lot easier than feeling worried or badly. I think that underneath you have the same sadness and frustration that I do about not being able to help him. I think we should figure out how to support each other, especially if we are ever going to figure out a way to help him.

Answer evaluation: Remember that answer **a** is not a correct assumption, and answers **b** and **c** are only satisfying thoughts in your head. Answer **d** puts the discussion back on course.

GIVE SUPPORT TO YOURSELF

Sources of support have to include yourself. To enhance your ability to be good to yourself look at how you handle your feelings, relationships, and diabetes under a microscope for a while. One way this can be done is by journaling. The writing seems to tap a part of the brain that is not used enough and helps you understand your personal feelings. Journaling means you take the time to actually sit down and observe yourself. The type of writing done in a journal is different from other writing you may have done. This writing is not for others. In fact, you don't need whole sentences or correct grammar. It is not to be judged.

A process similar to journaling is writing on-line. To write something down is to change the way you think about it. Seeing your thoughts become visible allows you to realize them in a profound way. To write to those you know using e-mail is a way of connecting with other people without seeing their reactions, feeling freer to express yourself without that feedback. For people who may not join a traditional support group because of shyness, limited mobility, or transportation problems, chat rooms in cyberspace or e-mailing a person on one of the various web sites might feel more comfortable and satisfactory. Here's another opportunity to identify with other people who have diabetes. A great place to begin is the American Diabetes Association's website at www.diabetes.org.

READING

Reading is a great source of support. There are many exciting and helpful books and magazines available to you, and new ones are coming out every day! Check in your local library or browse the bookstores. Contact the American Diabetes Association for their book list at (800) ADA-ORDER or 232-6733. The number to call for general diabetes information is (800) DIABETES or 342-2383.

THERAPY

Support can come from a relationship with a professional psychologist, social worker, psychiatrist, psychiatric nurse, or counselor (master's degree or doctorate) who specializes in chronic illness, stress management, behavioral or family therapy. Self-help or support groups are also good sources.

Positive reinforcement from inside yourself is important no matter where else you get support.

The Changing Nature of Families

They come in all sizes, shapes, and descriptions—traditional, single parent, dual career, blended, alternative, and makeshift. With awareness and education, we can balance our emotions through all the changes a family experiences. A family that functions well considers the mental and physical well-being of each person in the family. A family that doesn't work well is going to affect your diabetes control.

Nancy is 17-year-old girl who has had diabetes for 8 years. Understandably her family responded to her diagnosis with patterns of overinvolvement, overprotection, and inflexibility. They were not aware of how their behavior affected Nancy. She felt guilty that her diabetes had upset them greatly. She became enmeshed in their feelings about the diabetes—their fears and worries—and she was unable to get in touch with her own feelings. She felt sorry for her parents, not herself.

There was no place for her to cry out about her sadness, fears, or anger at having diabetes. Her parents had watched over her closely and advised her, and she had depended com-

pletely on them. She was afraid to do anything without them. Their well-meaning overprotection had made her feel like a much younger child than she actually was. Their initial response to her diabetes had never developed to the point of encouraging her to express her feelings and adjust so that she could set her own goals for life and diabetes management. Her parents did not experience her as rebelling; she was just depressed and withdrawn. Then she started to skip shots and meals, and her family became very upset with her when they could no longer control her.

When I met Nancy, she was visibly depressed in her demeanor, had no energy, and was underweight. She did poorly at school, never slept over at a friend's house, was disinterested in getting a driver's license, and her diabetes was way out of control. At first the family resisted therapy, feeling burned out and not wanting to put any more energy into her. They felt helpless and furious with her. Their anger turned to coldness. What felt to Nancy like emotional abandonment frightened her and deepened her depression.

Nancy also felt safe enough to open up about her feelings. She was afraid to grow up and have to take care of diabetes on her own. Therapy was a place where she was not afraid that she was burdening anyone. Gradually, working as a couple, the parents learned to respect the necessary boundaries of what they could do for Nancy and to speak of their concerns first with each other. As a team, they were able to listen to and accept the anger and anxiety that Nancy was learning to express in her therapy sessions, without getting depressed, too. Beginning to see themselves as separate from each other, they could untangle the enmeshed feelings. Using the skill of positive reframing, they could view Nancy's surprising fury as an opening to trust and healing for Nancy and the family. The therapy, combined with the medical team's teaching Nancy how to take care of herself, worked.

FAMILIES—HELP OR HINDRANCE

The ways of healthy families are the same for all families, with or without a chronic illness. Having diabetes in a family, however, intensifies the need for a family to work well together. There are several key components to well-balanced families.

1. One of the best predictors of success for an adult is being raised in a family that worked well together.
2. Feeling unconditionally loved as a child is a great part of the necessary positive framework. This means that despite your behaviors or the consequences your parents or society apply to them, your family still loves you for who you are. This concept is an ideal, not a constant state.
3. Predictable rules and predictable warmth, love, and closeness are vital to making a family work. Healthy families are in the process of balancing the conflicting energies of individuality—in roles, independence, and group closeness. For example, you can be close to your mother and still want to do things differently from her, to be a separate person.
4. Flexibility and resilience in feelings, behaviors, and tasks are also themes that run through happy families.

If you read this list and find yourself and your family faring poorly, don't despair. Yes, your first family—the family you came from—can be crucial as the healthy springboard that catapults you into your healthy family as an adult. However, if you did not grow up in a family with positive forces, that does not mean that you are doomed to fail or even repeat the negative patterns of your childhood. There is strong evidence of "resilient" children who turn out okay, despite all the limitations.

INSIGHT FROM THE PAST

Examining your past experiences and present expectations about how a family should be is helpful. Family matters, but you can create a good marriage. You can overcome those influences of the past through awareness, effort, good habits, and setting priorities. The following is an example of how old family interaction patterns create current family problems.

When Molly was diagnosed with diabetes as a child, her family separated her from the rest of the family. They treated her differently, delicately, and expected less from her in everything from family chores and what foods she could eat to school and social experiences. Molly needed acceptance rather than protection.

Molly was obsessed about getting away from her sickly, unloved perception of herself. In her 10 years of marriage, Molly never let her husband Mike help her with her diabetes. She was determined not to call attention to herself or her diabetes. She would slip out of bed quietly in the middle of the night to take care of her low blood glucose, intent on not letting him know what she was doing. Likewise, when her blood glucose sometimes went low after sex, she would run to the refrigerator, never telling him what she was doing. Mike, unaware of the true reason for this behavior, found her evasive and distant at those times. He felt frustrated by what seemed to him as detachment and coldness.

Molly's increased self-awareness and communication with her husband could work to challenge the power of the past and create a different, more positive experience for both of them in the present. (See chapter 3 on coping.)

Mike will see that Molly's behavior is not a rejection of him but rather an automatic reaction to her past. Mike will at least be able to understand her behavior, and he won't feel so disappointed.

UNCONDITIONAL LOVE IN ACTION

All children benefit from their family accepting them despite any imperfections, mistakes, or disappointments. This unconditional love does not ignore negative or disappointing behaviors but acknowledges them and continues to support and love the child. A family with this kind of love also has consistent discipline. There are predictable consequences for the child's actions.

> **HEALTHY FAMILIES**
>
> 1. Unconditional love
> 2. Family is a high priority
> 3. Predictable rules and expectations
> 4. Parents in charge
> 5. Encourage individuality
> 6. Interdependent
> 7. Flexibility
> 8. Regular and effective communication meetings
> 9. Forgiveness
> 10. A place for fun

In reality, unconditional love is a difficult concept. When it comes to adult relationships, it is harder still, and controversial. Sometimes adults can and perhaps should be "conditional" and decide to separate from their partners in the event of danger to the children or themselves. A partner or parent may excuse or ignore self-destructive behavior of a family member. This is called *enabling* him or her to continue that behavior. Enabling is different from unconditional love, which requires acknowledgment of the negative behavior. It is important to accept the person but to set limits on acceptance of certain behaviors.

When you don't commit to self-care over a long period, your partner or parent can get disheartened. What can they do, when you don't even try to acquire the knowledge, discipline, or self-esteem necessary for diabetes management? This is true for people who don't have diabetes, too. People are more attractive when they have a healthy lifestyle like the one required in diabetes. You also feel good about yourself when you are fit, exercising, and eating well.

Don was an alcoholic who also had diabetes. His wife always made excuses for his pressures in life and felt a little resentment toward the medical team for adding to the strain. She was not an ally in the team's efforts to get Don healthy. He had refused to go to counseling and AA meetings. The physicians were trying to get him to sign a contract with them about what he needed to do in his care. Finally, his wife broke the deadlocked negotiations and agreed to attend Al-Anon meetings with her children.

She began to realize that she had grown up with an alcoholic father and had coped by tolerating his behavior, thinking it was normal. After many months, she understood that she and her children did not have to live with her husband's alco-

holism. She told him that it was his choice whether to attend AA meetings. However, although she loved Don and would be heartbroken not to be married to him, she was not going to subject herself or the children to life with an alcoholic. He refused to go to the meetings.

She and the children left him for 6 weeks. When he started the AA meetings, she agreed to come home. Don was furious at the medical team for instigating all of this, at first. The doctors were interested in understanding his anger. The family's acknowledgment of their pain was the prelude to him beginning to take care of himself.

When you have diabetes, you need your family no matter how you mess up your control of the illness. You want them to root for you continually. You want a loving reaction, not a critical one, when you are not doing well. Yet, if you are the parent, spouse, or sibling without diabetes, it is hard to be more loving or to put in more effort when you are concerned or worried or angry at the person with diabetes for not taking care of him or herself.

Adults with diabetes can try to base love for their partners on the condition that they do not discuss diabetes at all. Giving and getting unconditional love and avoiding manipulation are important for you and your family. It is important to find approaches that provide the affection and cohesion that are essential for keeping the family together and promoting the changes that need to take place in self-management of diabetes. It may be difficult to change your orientation from the habit of anger to warmth and acceptance (for parents, spouses, and children).

One family balked at my suggestion that they hug their younger child, Laura, every time she had a tantrum. Part of their reaction was due to the difficulty in shifting out of anger. The other was not wanting to reward negative behavior. In this particular family, Laura's sister Alice had just been diagnosed with diabetes. Laura seemed to have a tantrum every time she needed some attention. I encouraged the family to look at the behavior from Laura's perspective. Then they could shift their focus to one of respect for her ability to try to get what she needed. ***(positive reframing)*** *The family needed to look at Laura's situation with love and compassion, not judgment.*

Laura and her parents made a pact that for 1 week, every outburst would be greeted by them sweeping her up into their arms. Laura could catch up on some of the attention that she felt she had lost. The week after that, Laura went back to having more self-awareness and control. The family was determined to make sure that she could get attention another way. She returned to feeling that she had a significant place in the family too and didn't need to be noticed for being in trouble. Positive changes that took an effort from each of them reminded Laura that she was loved and in a secure family setting.

MAKE THE FAMILY A TOP PRIORITY

The basic philosophical stance of unconditional love sets the stage. Next, we see that a family needs structure, communication, and leadership from the parents to keep it working. These are a natural result of individual, daily behaviors that lead to a "fit" family. Parents can go about family fitness in much the same way that you get and keep your body in shape. It requires first that the family be considered a top priority.

If your family is kept a priority, it can always be the healthy haven for renewing the energy you need to balance all the pressures in life. A family is a group of people you like who like you for both shared and differing goals. These are people who celebrate your joys with you and share the difficult parts of your life as well. Over a lifetime, you'll give energy to work, school, financial, physical, emotional, moral, and spiritual dimensions. Your family can be a source of nurturing that supports you and replenishes your energy in all the areas of your life. It is unfortunate that the family is often perceived as part of the drain on your energy. It does not have to be that way.

WHAT'S SO GREAT ABOUT RULES AND REGULATIONS?

A healthy family establishes rules, roles, and regularity. This just happens to fit in well with diabetes. The regularity comes from a structure of activities that make family members feel comfortable because they can be anticipated. There is peace when you can expect support, nurturing, communication, and consistent consequences to certain behaviors. Parents have to take the lead in maintaining order. Most teenage patients dislike the requirements—and consequences of not meeting them—set up by their parents. If asked privately, most adolescents are aware that they need protection as well as freedom. They also realize that their parents are helping them with their own limit-setting problems.

Predictable rules and nurturing in the family is similar to what Steven Covey *(The Seven Habits of Highly Effective Families)* is talking about when he refers to the "laws of the farm." He explains there is no way to make a farm successful without long-term problem solving and daily tending. There is no shortcut or catch-up to make crops grow or animals flourish. Families with diabetes need painstaking care. Without being regularly tended to, both diabetes and family life run into crisis after crisis. However, rules and structure are not more important than the emotional needs of each person in the family.

Melanie, who was 16 years old, would always beg her parents to drop the restrictions they applied after she defied their mutually-agreed upon rules about blood testing four times daily and logging it in her self-monitoring book, talked on the phone after hours, or was rude to her sister and parents. She would promise that she would be better. She went for the sympathy generated from her diabetes. It worked. Her parents would lower their standards, but that made them angry with her. Melanie always seemed delighted, at first, to get away with doing less.

In therapy, she unhappily noted the same pattern in her relationships with friends. She was letting them get away with not treating her well, much the same way her parents let her get away with not treating herself or them well. Melanie and her parents began to realize that the family climate and Melanie's relationships with her friends would only be helped by following through on the rules. Her parents feverishly read books on tough love and rehearsed scenarios with me to learn to say no with compassion. They spent time empathizing with Melanie on the difficulties of having diabetes and kept it separate from following through on the consequences of her behavior. They felt a renewed respect for their parenting, and Melanie liked having stronger role models to help her out with her friends. Of course, she was still snippy when her parents stuck to the rules, but they all had a better understanding of what was normal and healthy.

YOU ARE ALL INDIVIDUALS

In a family that is running well, every individual has a sense of personal power.

Fourteen-year-old Meg Smith had diabetes. Her father was preoccupied with trying to control Meg's eating and her blood glucose. He was indignant at her moodiness and deliberate skipping of blood sugar testing and insulin injections during school hours. He often said that he would never have shown such disrespect to his own father's rules. He felt badly about himself because he could not get her to do the right things.

The shift Mr. Smith had to make was to place equal value on Meg's feelings and thoughts. Before his wishes and commands could be respected, he had to really hear and empathize with Meg's fears and concerns. He told me that the therapist they had seen before blamed him for what was happening with Meg. At that point, he pulled the whole family out of therapy. He was angry that the other therapist had not shown him understanding or respect.

I listened and tried to show him that he and his daughter were having a similar experience. Neither he nor Meg was ever going to take any advice or direction until they felt recognized and validated for their feelings.

The parallel between his feelings toward the therapist and his daughter's feelings toward him made sense to Mr. Smith. He knew he had to drop his goals of making Meg listen to him and do what he wanted. He was going to listen to her first. So much is going on inside children, and parents do have to concentrate on how to make that shift and respect children's feelings by listening to them.

Mr. Smith did a great job. He dropped his commands and fear mongering. ("You know what will happen to you if you don't take care of yourself.") He tried to understand by asking questions in a sincere and interested manner. Meg was so relieved to open up to him. She too felt depressed and worried about the uncontrolled blood glucose. The lunch period was so short that she did not have time to break away from her friends to go to the bathroom to check and take her shot. She was skipping lunch because all her friends did. Anyway she was afraid to eat because she was not taking her lunchtime shot. She felt self-conscious about eating in front of others. Now, especially, she did not want to eat in front of others because she had begun to feel fat. When she got home from school, she would be starved and eat anything she could find in the house. The overeating left her with a distorted sensation of feeling stuffed and fat. As a result of these binges, she had gained weight. Meg broke into tears. Her dad held her for a long time.

He was upset with his own narrow vision of what she had to do to be a good girl. All of her behaviors made sense in the context of her feelings. "I am so happy you told me these things. You have had so much on your mind. I was wrong not to be there for you. I can see that some of our goals are the same. And I was missing what was stopping you from getting there." He was touched with her trust and delighted that he could relieve her loneliness and share her burdens. "I would be so pleased if you will continue to trust me with your feelings. I know I can help you."

Meg felt happy to have a partner. "Not so fast, Daddy," she joked. Now they had a shared perspective for problem solving diabetes issues. He was going to have to remember and use the listening and questioning skills to elicit his child's feelings. It wasn't that hard. He really did want to know them. His anxiety about her health and his responsibility in it had blocked his sensitivity. Fortunately, they were beginning to understand the problem underlying her behavior. This would give her a new way to deal with the social, body image, and eating issues.

Families can help us be healthy, productive, honest, loyal, loving, and loved—no matter what age we are. Alan Cohen says, in *The Dragon Doesn't Live Here Anymore*, that "the main thing is to keep the main thing, the main thing." This means that we need to honor whatever we decide is really important to us—our family, our health—no matter what outside forces, new challenges, moods, or events may threaten us.

HOW DO YOU MOTIVATE AN INDIVIDUAL?

Shame and embarrassment are not good motivators in health care, unless you want anger and conflict. Respect and caring about the individual come first. Good diabetes health care efforts can follow.

Harry, age 70, married to Delores, age 65, with type 2 diabetes, wants to yell at her for overeating and secret binges. This is the second marriage for both of them, and they have been blissfully happy for 7 years. He does not want to lose her. He is frightened by what he reads about complications. More important, Harry is impatient that Delores is always tired and irritable after her excessive eating and high blood glucose.

By extending tenderness to her and a desire to understand, Harry may be able to get her to go see a dietitian and a mental health specialist to understand what is triggering this new behavior. It may be that her eating patterns have changed to help her cope with some new worries. (Her son has recently been divorced, and the grandchildren don't seem to be returning her calls.) Harry must figure out a way to avoid trying to control her and being judgmental or angry. Together, with some professional help, they can discuss other healthier behaviors that might meet her needs.

It is a real challenge for families to preserve individual independence and yet share interests and concerns.

Stan, age 65, with type 2 diabetes for 25 years, came into his diabetes specialist's office with his wife, Dora, to whom he had been married for 40 years, for a routine visit. During the examination, the physician learned of Stan's sexual dysfunction. Improved diabetes control can sometimes be a solution, depending on the causes of the impotency. In Stan's case, the impotency was probably not going to be reversible through improved diabetes control. The doctor referred him to a urologist to discuss treatment possibilities, including a surgical penile implant.

Their marriage had been stormy for all but the last 10 years, coinciding with Stan's impotency problems. Dora was sexually abused as a child, which had affected her attitudes toward having sexual relations with her husband. She was anxious and depressed, before Stan began experiencing sexual functioning problems, when she anticipated his sexual approach. In response, he was angry and insulted and would put her down for the insult that he was feeling. When Stan was unable to achieve or maintain erections, Dora no longer feared him and became tender and loving toward him. Their relationship was the best it had ever been. They had maintained a positive and high level of intimacy for the last 10 years. They did better together when sexual intercourse was not a part of their lives. Dora then felt comfortable being sexual, knowing it would not end in intercourse.

Stan wanted the opportunity to be able to have intercourse again, and, of course, Dora needed respect for her fears. Here was an example of individual needs in a couple clearly coming into conflict.

After intensive counseling, Stan was willing to give up frequency and spontaneity—reframing it as planned anticipation—in exchange for the continued warmth and intimacy they were sharing. This resolution came about only because they made great efforts in therapy and at home learning how to really listen to each other and respect each other's needs.

INTERDEPENDENCE MEANS SHARING THE LOAD

Balancing work, diabetes, and other roles is complicated. You can be more effective in these areas by becoming **interdependent** with your family rather than focusing only on yourself.

John, the father of Peter, age 16, with diabetes, developed stress-related pains in his chest. His doctor gave him a prescription for some regular and intensive exercise. He felt overwhelmed by yet another obligation, this time for himself. He was still reeling from Peter's diagnosis and a need to comfort him and the whole family. His wife had criticized him for being preoccupied and detached from the children. It seemed that many situations, all at once, needed his problem solving.

He told Peter that he really admired how Peter had incorporated exercise into his life after he was diagnosed with diabetes. He needed Peter's help now to solve his own adherence problem. His solution was to ask his son to help him with his own difficulty with incorporating exercise into his daily life. John was figuring out a way to strengthen his relationship with his son and improve both their health. At the same time, he knew his relationship with his wife would benefit because she would be relieved about his health and pleased that he was reaching out to their son.

PLAN TO BE FLEXIBLE

Because of the ongoing nature of diabetes and the surprise events that occur in life, a family must use a flexible approach to diabetes. You can try to be orderly about when meals are eaten, who makes them, or who helps with the shots. But things will happen. People get sick, burnout, have to travel for work. People with diabetes run out of insulin, forget to test, or have unexpectedly low or high blood glucose. People are human.

FAMILY MEETINGS

One way to preserve family closeness is to provide one-on-one time for each individual in addition to some form of family meeting together, such as dinner, dessert, or before bedtime. Family meetings are a time for clarifying and prioritizing needs and goals. You can also address the problems that need to be solved and outline responsibilities, consequences, rewards, and desired outcomes. This is good in any family. For your family, it is especially necessary to communicate regularly, because diabetes brings more responsibility to each member.

The idea of meeting regularly allows the family to recognize and work on negative cycles or patterns that aren't working and find positive ways of relating to each other on the issues.

This includes individual contact, the physical warmth of touching and hugging, and the communicated positive reflections of each others' behavior or character.

There are so many tasks for a family to clarify with one another in diabetes management. For example, who makes the meals; monitors blood glucose; supervises exercise, low blood glucose, and healthful eating patterns; suggests insulin supplements; gives encouragement; aids in problem solving; and, depending on the age or situation, decides who gives shots? These roles need to be balanced, and both parents and siblings need to be involved so that no one is left out, burns out, or feels overwhelmed. Everyone should get positive reinforcement in the form of praise and incentives for all the work and effort that goes into making diabetes and the family run smoothly.

You must recognize that efforts at good diabetes care do not always result in good diabetes control. It takes tremendous patience sometimes to deal with this fact. That is why efforts rather than outcomes should be rewarded. The goal is to do your personal best and learn how to problem solve.

HURTS AND FORGIVENESS

Diabetes offers many opportunities for mistakes and hurts. This makes the family even more important as the place to learn the healing principle of forgiveness. You don't want to let either the intentional or unintentional misunderstandings or mistakes of others have the power to hurt you for too long. You do not want your behavior to injure others. In healthy families, forgiveness can come more easily because there is a general sense of trust and mutual respect.

The power of forgiveness is evident in 21-year-old Paulette's feelings about her low blood glucose experiences. For Paulette, low blood sugars meant she was out of control, because she had done something wrong. She felt like a failure and was ashamed of those experiences. The family had, perhaps, contributed to her judgmental, critical opinion of herself. They would respond with alternating reactions of anger or pity for what Paulette called her mistakes. Their interactions reinforced Paulette's negative self-beliefs. The family felt badly both about how they behaved and felt and about how Paulette was behaving and felt about herself.

What challenged this ongoing interaction pattern happened with her new boyfriend, Mark. He was with her one day when she had a low blood glucose reaction. For him, needing to take over temporarily and help her with her blood glucose made him feel even more intimate with her. He saw her vulnerability, what she described as her "bare essence" when they had talked about it later. He felt close, loving, and happy to share something so personal with her. He felt strong and trusted. For him, the low blood glucose reaction was neither frightening nor something to be judged. She merely needed assistance, and he was there to support her.

Mark began the conversation about how moved he felt being able to play such an important part in her life. Paulette was embarrassed and put herself down during the discussion. He was shocked at her response. He challenged her long and hard about how she and her family were looking at this. Paulette had no choice but to look at how she had felt for so long about her experiences with having low blood glucose. This involved forgiving herself and her family for the critical way they had been behaving. With information that Mark found, he realized that the low blood glucose resulted from her efforts to be in good health. He told her that, even if it happened many times, he hoped to see it in the same light. "If it was from carelessness or poor planning," he wondered out loud, "why would I judge you for your humanness?"

He confronted her with her own misconceptions. His positive perception changed Paulette's understanding. She was forced to rethink her opinion of herself. This, in turn, led her to respond differently to her family's criticisms that no longer fit her. She began to challenge them. They were happy to look at these interactions differently too. There had been too much unnecessary hostility in the past.

CONSIDER CULTURAL INFLUENCES

Sometimes, the strength of the intergenerational support system can work in reverse.

Cary, an African American grandmother with type 2 diabetes, was in the role of taking care of her daughter and her grandchildren in her home. Cary described herself as nervous from the pressures and the noises of the younger children. She felt she had priorities other than taking care of her health, which would mean paying attention to her diet and exercise. When she was asked to come in to address this problem, Cary's daughter Adrienne was relieved.

Adrienne had wanted to move out on her own but did not want to embarrass or abandon her mother. Their separation would allow them to enjoy each other more, while giving Adrienne the responsibilities she was happy to have. Cary could then concentrate on the foods that were better for her health and enjoy a more stress-free, enhanced quality of life. Cary could remain the family matriarch from her separate household. Her grandchildren could enjoy the benefits of a very involved but healthier grandmother.

Often with first-generation immigrants, the children operate as go-betweens for medical information needed in their parent's medical care. Authority is passed from the parents to the children. This can make the parents feel childlike, even rebellious, and less likely to assume direct responsibility for their health. It also takes a toll on the children, giving more responsibility than necessary for their age and role. When the child has diabetes and the parents cannot communicate with health care providers, except through the children, it is doubly difficult for the parents to supervise their child's health.

LAUGH AND THE FAMILY LAUGHS WITH YOU

Families should enjoy each other. Using humor is helpful in most interactions. Being able to laugh at yourself and laugh about conflicts or differences is crucial. Humor—even about the tough stuff—is a coping skill you can acquire. Trying to appreciate and preserve your children's sense of humor may pay off in the long run. Humor levels in a family can and will improve with concentration and practice.

Parents of Children with Diabetes

Over the course of a lifetime, there will be many times that one or another family member will need to express the frustrations and worries of living with a chronic disease. As parents, you may feel resentment, jealousy, anxiety, guilt, fear, and depression at the diagnosis and again at later stages of your child's growth. If you don't recognize and express these feelings, you may find yourselves stuck in frustrating patterns.

As you read the chapters in this book, you learn about feelings other parents and children have had in your situation and ways to express your feelings in satisfying ways for yourself and other family members. All of your children—with and without diabetes—need to learn to cope with strong feelings, such as the ability to comfort themselves when they feel sad or afraid and to set limits on their own behavior. You do, too.

THE SAME OLD SKILLS

The skills involved in taking care of diabetes are the same skills used to make a marriage work well or to raise

EXERCISES

Parent to parent: Your husband says he can't believe you let your son's blood sugars go so much out of line. Your response to your husband depends on whether you give yourself time to allow your feelings to surface, respect yourself for feeling them, and take a moment to understand them. Your response might be:

1. "That's easy for you to say. You do nothing to help."
2. "It is just one more area I feel terrible about."
3. "I am speechless that you said that."
4. "I know you are as upset as I am, so I will try to forgive you for that comment. We are in this together. We have to be careful not to blame each other or our child. Our focus has to be on figuring out why there was such a drastic change and then we need to come up with some possible remedies."

ANSWER EVALUATION

1. This is aggressive and won't lead to mutual support or problem solving.
2. This reinforces your bad feeling about yourself. Nothing is accomplished, however. You've missed the point that your son needs help in his diabetes control, and you need support from your spouse.
3. This response is honest and effective because you *pause* rather than react. It expresses anger and shock. **(ventilation)** This gives your partner time to think about what he said and perhaps apologize or begin to face his own anxiety about his son's well-being.
4. This is a strong and competent answer. You are going out of your way **(empathy)** to get some comfort from your husband and some teamwork. **(persistence)** Understanding that your spouse is human, and hostile, at times when he is frightened or feeling guilty is important. Your generosity sets the stage for an eventual apology.

EXERCISES

Parent to child: Your child with diabetes, age 12 and entering a new school, tells you there is no way she will wear her diabetes alert bracelet in public. Again, pause to become aware of all the feelings this brings up in you. Your response might be:

1. "Oh yes, you will. I am the parent here. I happen to know best."
2. "You know what can happen to you if you don't."
3. "I am glad you are telling me what your plans are. Your openness with me on these personal matters is important." **(positive assertion)**
4. "What feelings brought you to this decision? **(assertive request)** Dad and I would really like to understand what you are thinking and feeling."

ANSWER EVALUATION

1. This is natural and easy to say. It is, however, aggressive and not very effective. You may be trying to wield power that you don't actually have. As your child grows up, you have less and less influence over what s/he does. You want to create in your child the ability to think and make decisions when you are not there.
2. Intimidation may work for a while, but it also creates anxiety and eventually backfires.
3. This is a **positive assertion,** taking time to reinforce what you are pleased about, that is, your child's communication with you. It can open a dialogue because you have shown respect for your child. After you do some good listening, it will be your time to voice your opinion.
4. This **assertive request** effectively elicits information so that you can respond to your child's real concerns rather than responding to your best guess about his/her motives. (No mind reading allowed.) By doing this, you can avoid the lecturing posture, which is guaranteed to bring about the famous eyeball rolls, blank stares, or cries of "Oh, Dad!!"

EXERCISES

Child to parent: All of your girlfriends have started having sleepovers at each other's homes. Your parents tell you they don't think you are ready to do that. You feel anger, surprise at being so mistrusted, annoyance, and maybe a bit relieved—you are worried about the responsibility, too. Your response might be:

1. "I hate you. You are the worst parents."
2. Nothing, but think about ways you can get them back secretly.
3. Nothing, but go to the pantry and pull out a handful of cookies.
4. "I understand that you are saying no because you think that is what you are supposed to do to be a good parent. **(assertive empathy)** I think this is overprotection. It makes me afraid to do new things, too. It makes me resent you and my diabetes."

ANSWER EVALUATION

1. You are expressive but not clear.
2. Uh oh. Dangerous. Better to show them how their fears (and yours) are understandable but unfounded.
3. Bad for your mental health and your blood sugar level. You need to learn to cope in ways that get good results.
4. **Assertive empathy** keeps your parents from feeling defensive. Sharing your feelings first can open the conversation that you need to have. Both children and parents like to come up with solutions rather than being told what to do. This will be a good start to addressing their fears (and yours) so you can sleep over. Health care professionals can add insight and reassurance for you and your parents about how normal this situation is and help you plan ahead and make good decisions. You might first have to say, "I am feeling too upset to talk. I will cool down and talk to you later."

a healthy family. Remember that if one person makes the conscious choice to practice good communication, there will eventually be a change in how the other person responds or interacts, too. Be persistent. Sometimes the patterns of poor interaction are so ingrained that when you change, the receiving party cannot really hear you at first.

WHY BOTHER?

You will be relieved that you have expressed your feelings, made your point, and not lost your temper, stayed depressed, or begun to overeat. You create the opportunity for the other person to feel better, be closer to you, and best of all, talk to you in a way that makes you feel more comfortable, too. Dr. Alan Jacobson's study at the Joslin Diabetes Center found that the group of children who had the worst glucose control over 4 years were from families who were not close and did not have open discussions. Better communication and closeness within families not only feels good emotionally but has a profound effect on blood glucose control.

Remember as you try new communication skills that it takes patience to stick with them and to see a difference. You must stand your ground, remembering that you may need to repeat your new endeavors. Keep your sense of humor. Even as you become more skillful in communicating, don't be thrown off by old behaviors—yours or anyone else's. (See chapter 3 on coping.)

MODELING BEHAVIOR

The most important reason to communicate as well as you can is that your children are listening to you. You are their role models, and from you they inherit attitudes about themselves, diabetes, food, and blood glucose levels. It is both exciting and frightening that your children listen so closely and will copy or rebel against your view of diabetes. The conversations that your children hear between you will be the same ones they play over in their heads and will be similar to the conversations they have with you. If you criticize each other, you probably also criticize your child. The voice that your child takes in and uses for himself will probably be a critical one, too.

We were doing role-plays. John called his wife, Emily, to find out what their 5-year-old Alice's predinner blood sugar level was. Emily was already angry, anticipating his nightly call, where the first thing was always the hateful blood sugar question. She hated that he seemed to check up on her, as if she could not take care of their daughter's diabetes. He never asked about how she was doing. Even worse was that she often felt like lying to her husband about the results. He would snap at her when the blood sugars were not in the normal range, which was often. "What did you do? Why is she 300?"

Freeze this picture. It is 10 years later. This time the questioning is not from spouse to spouse but from Emily to 15-year-old Alice. Alice is angry and evasive. Five years later, when Alice is on her own, the voice in her head about handling her diabetes is critical and demanding. Ten years later, Alice will have similar conversations with her husband.

As I was listening to conversations of the parents managing their children's diabetes, I realized that they were the same conversations I had heard for years from adults with diabetes. It seems very obvious. How often do kids dread the inevitable question, "Did you test?" It only reminds them that they didn't. One more negative to put into their self-esteem pile. How often do they feel like lying to their parents about test results because the parents get all bent out of shape, making everyone uncomfortable? The conversations were frighteningly familiar.

PARENTS AS A TEAM

So, let's start at the source. If parents can learn to work as a team, helping one another, that will filter down to the children. It is a basic parenting fact that children watch and copy us, for better or for worse. With lots of laughter and repeated attempts shared with the group, John and Emily toiled at trying to have a good conversation. Before role-playing for the group, they talked about their feelings, to understand why they both react the way they do.

Emily, a perfectionist, gets burned out and feels guilty about unreal expectations for her 5 year old. She sits crying softly. Diabetes is still new and painful, and she cannot imagine letting go of the despair. John, and the other fathers, talk about how diabetes makes them feel. They describe feeling helpless, out of control, imperfect as parents, and a loss of pride. John feels like a defective father and a failure because he can't protect his family. He says that perhaps he deserved this because he had not originally been excited when his wife told him she was pregnant. He appears relieved to get this out as the tears roll down his cheek. The entire group is teary-eyed, feeling empathy for him and the similarities in their own lives.

John understands that he snaps at Emily because he feels guilty about not being there to help and protect them. He is also working on handling the additional financial pressures that diabetes brings. He feels disappointed that diabetes has curtailed his wife's going back to work, for now. This changes their financial planning and frustrates her personal need to go back to her career. It is easier for him to be irritable and critical than it is to face his own pain. He is really judging himself, not his wife, but it is easier to jump on her to get out his frustration.

John vows that he will try to think first and not react. It will be difficult for him to change this pattern. For Emily, the only behavior that she can control is her own. She comes up with a plan to stop and redirect the conversation so John can move toward being the helpful husband he would like to be.

John: I am calling to find out how your day has been. I would be happy to help you with any diabetes frustrations or decision making.
Emily: It's nice to hear from you. I have had a really good day. I am trying not to let the high blood sugar levels make me feel guilty and anxious. I know they are just numbers. I am glad to be honest with you. I know you can talk me out of feeling badly, and we can try to understand together why they might be high and what to do to get them down.
John: When you talk like that I feel calm, too. Thanks. Have I told you lately that I love you?

The group laughs at how artificial this sounds. They agree that contrived has to come before natural and is a far cry from the disagreeable ways they had been talking to each other before rehearsing new communication patterns.

COMMUNICATION PROCESS

Practice, practice, practice. First you recognize the feelings. Then you express them. Then you validate the feelings. Listen to your partner without feeling it is an attack on you. Just listen. Put compassion in the mix for yourself and others and, presto, you have better feelings, interactions, and even better diabetes care—something that money cannot buy.

WHOM DO YOU TELL?

One father in the group spoke of not wanting to tell others about his son's diabetes. He and his wife were forever arguing because she wanted to be open and tell everyone so they could help protect her son and to rid herself and her son of feeling embarrassed about keeping it a secret. Many of the fathers, valuing independence, agreed that they wanted their children to be private about their diabetes, fearing that the children would be treated differently.

This issue comes up again between parents and older children about who and when to tell. It is the same issue that young adults have in their heads when they are dating, who and when to tell that they have diabetes. There is not one right answer. But however it is done, we cannot sacrifice the goals of emotional and physical well-being. This issue must be discussed in families, with everyone having a say—including the siblings, who have needs, too—to come to a decision about what is safe and emotionally comfortable.

FRIENDSHIP

We know from research and observation that your children's major source of social support, toward the end of elementary school and through adolescence, are their peers. With this in mind, it seems obvious that friends ought to be part of the diabetes experience. However, Dr. Jacobson's research on newly diagnosed children with diabetes suggested that 55% of them did not discuss diabetes with their friends and another 35% thought they would be more likable without diabetes. These children don't realize that being open about diabetes can add to their self-esteem and being accepted by others.

Dr. Annette LaGreca's research suggests that families and the medical team should encourage openness with friends, and give friends diabetes education. After all, home away from home for adolescents is their peer group.

BOYS AND GIRLS

Most adolescent girls have a higher level of emotional support from friends than boys do. However, it appears that adolescent girls have more episodes of diabetic ketoacidosis and hospitalizations than males. It is not understood why that is, but possibly there are biological reasons or behavioral reasons such as less exercise or body-image issues. If friends are educated about good diabetes care, they may be able to help your teenager avoid these serious episodes.

Fortunately, being competitively athletic and proud of your body has a direct connection with well-controlled diabetes and a positive self-image. Boys' athletic activity, generally higher than girls', may account for their better metabolic control. Olga Silverstein, a family therapist who wrote *The Courage to Raise Good Men*, voices concern that in our society, we teach boys to be strong by denying and not sharing feelings. Strength may look like independence but perhaps it is merely isolation. This leaves boys more at risk emotionally and physically. Their feelings can be expressed through healthy physical activity, but they can also be acted out through reckless behaviors or bodily stress.

Adolescent girls without diabetes have more anxiety than adolescent boys. This underscores our need to assess and treat anxiety and depression before expecting the child to improve metabolic control.

It is easier to take care of diabetes with openness. I have seen an individual with an open, natural acceptance of diabetes inspire that acceptance in friends, school, and work so that other people have the same comfortable reaction.

ROLES DIABETES DICTATES

Children will take on roles in the family as needs dictate. Flexibility in these roles and having more than one is important.

Joe, a handsome 15-year-old with diabetes, was a positive, successful, athletic honor student. His memory of his diagnosis of diabetes was that everyone around him was crying. He wondered what he did to hurt them like that. He remembered not having any of his own feelings but being in tune with having sympathy for everyone else.

The medical team discovered his repressed anger and fears toward the diabetes when it showed up in a conversation where he revealed he didn't want to have children. The team was shocked and saddened to hear him say this. Along with his family, they had been a bit too proud of how positive he was. Joe felt forced to contain his bad feelings, to keep his family and medical team happy. Unable to express his anger, he had turned it on himself. He didn't like himself well enough to want to reproduce or feel that he deserved a full life. He didn't want the guilt of having a child with diabetes.

The conversation was a breakthrough for Joe. It allowed him to see that he and his family could accept his feelings, even if they weren't positive.

FINANCES

All members of the family need to address the financial issues that diabetes brings. You can get creative and involve yourselves with other families to find out the latest on cutting costs on medical supplies or insurance. Eating at home is often healthier and more economical. Healthier foods can be cheaper than packaged, high-fat, processed foods. Whereas buying in bulk is cheaper, it is easier for your children to take a serving size when they have access to individual servings. This means you have to plan ahead, and divide the goods into single servings. Parents may feel burdened and the children without diabetes may feel resentful of where the money goes, but the child with diabetes must not be made to feel at fault. The extra financial responsibility that diabetes brings is just a fact, not an emotionally charged liability. (See chapter 7 for more information on finances.)

LIFE STAGES OF CHILDREN

Diabetes over each of the life stages of a child—infant (0–2 years), toddler/preschooler (2–6 years), school-age child (6–12 years), adolescent (12–18 years), and young adult—brings particular challenges. Biological changes are matched with psychological and social changes as well. Just as there are different skills and tasks to be mastered in each period of growing up, so too, must the tasks of diabetes fit in. Knowing what is normal for each age is a great starting point for forming your expectations of how many diabetes self-care tasks your child can do.

There is no reason not to expect children with diabetes to be well adjusted. To help your child handle the emotional challenges of having diabetes through the life stages:

- You need a strong marital team and medical team.
- Befriend and share adventures with families with similar-aged children.
- Set healthy eating patterns for the entire family.
- Avoid using food as a reward or punishment.
- Stick to normal rules of parenting.

All parents struggle with learning to let go during various stages of their kids' growing up. Add diabetes and the challenge is multiplied. For parents of young children with diabetes, it is their diabetes too, in the beginning. Giving your child shots is probably a lot worse than giving yourself a shot. It fills you with emotional pain, greater than the physical pain the child is feeling.

Infants. With infants, you have to deal with the guilt of inflicting pain through shots and tests and trying to detect hypoglycemia, particularly at night, without direct assistance from your child.

Toddlers. In the toddler period, where language and mobility are part of the growing independence, your fear can make you overprotect and inhibit the child's healthy freedom. Guilt can make it difficult for you to set limits that are needed. Temper tantrums are sometimes difficult to distinguish from low blood sugars. At this age, kids are in tune with your emotional responses and relate them back to themselves. This makes it very important for you to be composed when you are explaining things. In this time of bounding imagination, play is an excellent outlet for toddlers and pre-school children to work out some of the fears (the pain and meaning of shots) diabetes brings to them that they cannot articulate with language.

School-aged. In the elementary school years, your child begins to fit into other environments and friendships. You need to put in extra effort to make life as normal as possible within the boundaries of good diabetes care. At the same time, you help your children accept the necessary differences in their behaviors so they can be comfortable with their peers, a requirement of this period. Kids need to feel unashamed about tasks such as eating snacks when others are not or checking blood glucose in the classroom in front of others or having to leave the room to do it. Gradually giving them diabetes tasks to be performed on their own (self-reliance), as they grow more curious and interested, is a way of boosting self-esteem. Make allowances for them not always following meal plans or checking blood glucose. This is normal, and your acceptance helps them deal with the moral (good and bad) issues of this time. Being able to tell you the truth about blood glucose results or other behaviors means that who s/he is and how s/he is doing is good enough for you. (See *Sweet Kids* by Richard Rubin and Betty Brachenridge, and *Ten Keys to Helping Your Child Grow up with Diabetes* by Tim Wysocki.)

Adolescence. Adolescence is in a class by itself, a time of upheaval emotionally, physically, and in diabetes control. It is the period of acute self-awareness, newly found responsibilities, and the need to experiment. In this period of children letting go of their childhood, you must take on new roles of guiding, and you must let go a little more—a difficult balance.

WHAT'S GOOD FOR THE KIDS

Psychologist Carol Dweck has suggested that it is better to praise efforts in learning rather than the results. She also found that giving credit for successful efforts rather than natural ability or intelligence motivated children to try new or more difficult things. This seems like good advice. Praise your children's efforts in taking care of their diabetes rather than focusing only on individual blood glucose readings. In the long run, verbal praise (and self-praise) is superior to concrete rewards, but external incentives are often important to get a child motivated. If your reinforcement is verbal, your children will more likely internalize the response and assume more responsibility for themselves as they mature physically and emotionally. The help and guidance of parents and authority figures should reinforce, not compete with, a child's confidence.

The concept of external rewards (often referred to as bribes) is very controversial because people fear that children may not value the task for itself. In diabetes, the goal would be for the child to take pride in his/her own efforts and actually begin to realize that s/he likes feeling better physically with more controlled blood glucose. One thing child development experts do agree on, though, is that what is expected from each of you in a system involving rewards must be clear and agreed on by both parent and child.

It is not always easy to do the right thing, even when you know what it is. We are all wrapped up in ratings and scores, an emphasis brought on by our culture, our competitive natures, and sometimes the medical team. Don't lose sight of the child and his/ her needs to be loved and respected in spite of the outcomes of blood glucose testing.

Other research cautions about the effects of parental overinvolvement on children. Dr. Cain, at Gettysburg College, worked with 3-year-old children and found that mothers who determinedly set high goals and pointed out mistakes had children who were easily caught up in shame responses (self-conscious, self-critical, and withdrawing behaviors) with even a hint of mother's disappointment. This might lead children to restrict and narrow their efforts or to give up too quickly. The issues here—overcontrol and standards that are not realistic—are a warning you must heed when supervising diabetes management for your children. It is natural for parents and physicians to get caught up in directing and judging. Out of necessity, you are constantly giving the child feedback. Unfortunately, this might have the effect of taking away the initiative for kids to want to do it on their own, or it may reduce their confidence. Diabetes management tasks are more likely to be completed when they are developed as personal empowerment.

There is so much imperfection in diabetes. You must help your children accept and adapt to the physical and emotional cycles that affect their lives and their blood sugar levels. They follow your lead. There are good honest efforts at care that do not result in equally good outcomes. Don't let your children try too hard to please you. You don't want them to feel ashamed of any parts of themselves.

WHEN THINGS GO WRONG

Ask your health care team to help you respect what you're doing so you can be more realistic and effective in achieving the balance of bringing up a happy well-rounded child who also happens to have diabetes. No easy task. Be proud of your efforts, too!

BACK TO NORMAL

Normal implies that you set limits and discipline the same way you would if your child did not have diabetes. Normally you would educate yourself in strategies and gain knowledge about each age group. If you are generally satisfied with your parenting and a special problem comes up with your child who has diabetes, ask yourself, "What would I do now if my child did not have diabetes?"

This is probably the most common story told in my office and in support groups.

Susan and Bob are the parents of Sara, a 7-year-old girl who has had diabetes since she was 3. Susan and Bob tell me they are having problems with Sara who now seems spoiled and manipulative. She has tantrums every time she is told to do something. At those times, Sara also complains that she does not feel well. Susan and Bob also seem distant from each other. Bob has no patience with Susan. Susan has no patience with Sara. Susan is often tired or preoccupied waiting for low blood glucose reactions. Bob feels neglected and resentful of his wife. They do not go out alone together. Everything is a family event. Susan claims there are no baby-sitters to be found. Bob snaps back at her that she won't look. Bob is intolerant of her anxiety about separating from her daughter. Bob and Susan have basically stopped having sex since the diagnosis of diabetes.

ALL PARENTS DO

The issues that are universal to all parents are setting limits for the children; developing a balance between discipline, expectations, and permissiveness; prioritizing time for parents' necessities and pleasures, and keeping authority for the parents only. These issues that all parents struggle over are intensified in families where a child has diabetes.

There is a fall from innocence the first time parents of a child who is newly diagnosed go from feeling love and compassion to the normal array of feelings in raising a child—exasperation, frustration, and even anger. No parent feels only love when raising a child. Parents who have a child with diabetes feel particularly guilty the first time they are furious with that child. The temptation to make the child center stage is exaggerated when a child has diabetes. The problem is that the family often does not then put diabetes in a normal place. Normal is when diabetes tasks are managed similar to other issues, such as doing homework or making the bed.

If you lower your expectations, you can create children who don't function up to their full potential. They can begin to appear as manipulative monsters rather than children who have accurately drawn conclusions about what they can get away with. In the case of Susan and Bob, I was impressed with the good job they have done with raising their daughter. Although she seems spoiled and controlling at home, Sara is very successful in taking care of her diabetes and in getting along with friends and enjoying school.

Isn't it amazing how tough parents are on themselves when the inevitable problems come up? Life is not about trying not to have problems. It is about recognizing them and showing resilience in finding solutions.

Susan agreed that she has difficulty following through with the consequences she had set for Sara's behavior. She was always sure she had overreacted and given out too harsh a punishment. She would begin to feel guilty that she had been angry with her child who had so much to go through because of the diabetes. She had unconsciously taught Sara that nagging, tantrums, or comments that she did not feel well could get her anything. This had repercussions for Sara—parental anger and resentment. They did not let her sleep at her friends' houses nor did they go out socially themselves. Sara often had stomach aches at transitional or separation times (separation anxiety). It would occur when she was going to her room to do homework, to take a bath, or to bed. She did not seem to like going off alone or leaving her parents by themselves.

The plan they came up with was to look behind the manipulation to find a need or a feeling such as anxiety that was being met in an unfortunate way. With this new thought in place, they could recognize Sara's behavior with a response of interest and compassion. They would ask her to describe the feeling. Next they would determine whether blood sugar needed to be checked. Finding normal blood sugars, the parents would repeat the direction, "Take your bath now," and add, "I will come in and spend time with you when you are ready for bed. I think you will be feeling better by then." This would be followed by a quick hug. In summary, the plan was to recognize their daughter's need, meet it briefly, repeat the instructions, and offer to provide other attention or problem solving later.

This new manner of reacting would teach Sara a new principle. It would show that her parents were in charge and that her needs would be acknowledged but not indulged until her required tasks were done. Most of the attention Sara needed would now be given for successful experiences. She would feel better for accomplishing her tasks and having interested parents who were not angry with her.

MEALTIMES

Battles over eating occur in many families. Solve the situations before they turn to war by using normal parenting rules. Go for normal behavior and expectations, even if your heart is not following your head. Remember it is normal to have children who are picky about eating or intent on only a few foods. There are, however, positive methods to fit diabetes control in with this. If your child plays with his food and dinner takes forever, what would you do if your child didn't have diabetes? Well then, do it. If it means that for your other children you set the timer and clear away the food at the bell, so be it. You may have to treat some low blood sugar reactions, but you will be less angry at your child. Normal is to have an enjoyable eating experience, focusing not only on the food but on the family. Remember, it never happens smoothly all the time in any family.

After you clean off the table, knowing your child has probably not eaten enough to last until snack time, take your irritated and broken heart into the bedroom. Take your spouse with you, set the timer for your anger, find comfort, and assign who will have the watchful eye for catching or preventing low blood glucose. It may come, of course, and you will be prepared. This action will help you avoid long-lasting preoccupation with food and negativity at mealtime, not to mention in relationships. Please discuss these ideas with your physicians, first, so that you have a plan that fits all possibilities.

THE PARENTAL TEAM

One of the basic tasks for any set of parents is learning how each can complement the other as they parent. Both parents must learn to handle all the tasks of diabetes management to prevent burnout and preserve freshness and flexibility in their approach to childrearing. If yours is a single-parent home, you need to find another adult who can learn to co-parent with you at times.

Kathy and Peter are the parents of 10-year-old Linda who has diabetes. On a day-to-day basis, Kathy does most of the blood testing and shots. On Saturdays, when Peter takes over, he and Kathy seem to have a regular fight when she gets home from her errands. Linda's blood sugar is usually higher than normal. The message that Kathy receives is guilt for going out and leaving Linda under Peter's care. For his part, Peter is demoralized knowing he can never do as good a job as Kathy. Frankly, he is hoping not to have the responsibility anymore, much as he enjoys being alone with his daughter. They usually fight enough to make them cancel the baby-

sitter they have for that one special date a week. Kathy is then secretly relieved because she feels that only she can get the blood sugars back down.

This scenario is painfully common. People live with unpleasant situations for such a long time, thinking there is no other way to remedy the feelings or the situation. To change this, it is helpful to reevaluate what their needs are and rewrite the meanings that each parent has assigned to the situation. Kathy does need the break. Peter does need the connection with his daughter. Kathy needs to nurture Peter's efforts, too, rather than getting upset about the outcome. With more experience and her support, he can learn to make more accurate decisions about the amount of insulin, choice of food, and what limits to set with his daughter. He needs to feel positive about spending time with and taking care of his daughter. He is at the stage experienced by many grandparents—feeling sorry for the limitations on the child and not feeling as though he wants to be the one to have the responsibility. If he faces up to his own feelings, he can move on to a more effective relationship with his child.

Often grandparents or a divorced and noncustodial parent is more lenient about all the rules that parents set up. Everyone prefers to be the good guy. The truly good person is the one who helps a child to be disciplined and organized. Sometimes part-time caretakers don't think they need to follow through in the same way—it's only for a day. With patience and coaching and positive reframing about how to put the time in, Peter would become intellectually and emotionally better prepared to handle his daughter's diabetes. He would benefit by feeling competent, and happy that he was a real partner to his wife, and look forward to a nice evening together. Kathy would have less guilt, some private time to take care of her needs, and look forward to a satisfying time with her husband. They both needed something from each other.

Sometimes it is hard to master a skill because you don't get to do it often enough. The father who only occasionally gives shots probably shakes each time. Remember, kids don't want to upset their parents. Seeing their parents upset about them reflects on how they view themselves. A parent who delivers the message that diabetes is too hard to deal with can make the child feel that they are too difficult to be around, too.

Children are smart, too, and will probably want to choose the parent who does the better job. It is important not to leave out one of the parents because of the child's reactions. Both parents can be equally competent caregivers. Even in diabetes, it is not healthy for children to be dictating to their parents—that's different from requesting and sharing feelings.

Shortly after he was diagnosed, Tony, age 6, screamed and said he did not want his father to give him shots. "Your shots hurt," he said. Have you ever seen a 35-year-old man revert to feeling like he was on the playground and wasn't picked for the team? That is exactly what Tony's father, Tom, felt. On top of that, he did not want to upset his son, who had enough to bear with the diabetes. Tom was devastated. He gave no more shots. His wife, Sue, became burdened by having no breaks. There was a tension between them. It was as if Sue was the favorite parent and Tom had stepped back and given up.

They are good parents and would have easily been able to discuss this and choose another reaction if the issue had not been about diabetes. Luckily, not too soon after this happened, they shared the problem in a support group. There were smiles and whispers as other parents acknowledged similar events in their families. We discussed that children needed to say why they preferred one parent to another, as a way of validating them and identifying what issues needed to be worked on.

They practiced saying, "I am glad you told me Mommy does it better. She is not the only person who will be giving you shots. Sometimes I will be giving them. I want you and Mommy to teach me to be as good, or even better. I don't want to be left out of being close to you and helping you to take care of your diabetes. Do you want to start tonight or tomorrow?"

This gave their child a choice that was more acceptable to them. It would be a relief to the child, in some ways, to have the parents back in control again. Controlling parents is only fun in the short run. Having both parents love you and not be angry or distant is much better.

SIBLING RIVALRY

Stay with your parenting instincts, don't change how things are managed because of the diabetes. This includes tolerating your children fighting. Children do learn skills through fighting. They figure out how to solve problems, know when to stop, recover, and move on. So often parents focus unnecessarily on getting their children to stop fighting. Instead, give more attention to noticing when they are resilient about arguments and when they do well together, playing, sharing, talking, and cooperating.

Being resented more than usual by an older or younger sibling can be damaging to your child's health. For your child's self-esteem to blossom, s/he needs the protection and admiration of brothers or sisters. You playing favorites destroys that opportunity. Sibling bonds are important to a child's identity. When you feel loved and enjoyed and chosen, you are more likely to grow up feeling worthwhile. You are hurting both children when you favor one, even if it is for a good reason like compensating for diabetes.

Diabetes should not drastically change the rules and expectations. For example, preschoolers may need more supervision when they are fighting with each other because they are still learning social skills, and teenagers less intervention so as not to intensify their competition. In the "in between" age, when children already have some social skills, it is probably a good idea to stand back and be a facilitator, not a referee. Leaving siblings on their own when they should be keeps the child with diabetes from becoming manipulative and increases opportunities for healthy independence.

You do not want to end up giving the message that your child will always need special attention or favors or less pressure from friends, teachers, sports, or work. That won't work if s/he wants success in any of those areas. Your child needs to learn to take the time to take care of him or herself and develop a hardy point of view when s/he is challenged. Your child's identity is as a person first, not as a diabetic.

GOING TO SCHOOL REGULARLY

One of the ways to help your children is to encourage them to keep their competence up in school. It is easy to relax the control you might take with a child who does not have diabetes and wakes up not feeling well. Not feeling well is vague, and children with diabetes may have the same anxieties that other children have about going to school, for example, a test, unfinished homework, or a bully. Again, use the normal guideline to determine whether you would allow your child without diabetes to stay home.

Your child's job, and hopefully pleasure, is going to school. Sometimes knowing that school is going to happen, no matter what, keeps a child from using diabetes, consciously or unconsciously, not to go to school. You can have empathy about them not feeling well, be firm about them going, and be positive about them feeling better soon. Frequent absenteeism that could result from many episodes of not feeling well leaves a child behind and feeling different. In no way do we want that message given to our children or their friends or teachers. As adults, they will want to have staying power and do their best.

PLAYING SPORTS

The same is true for keeping your child's sense of self positive in the area of athletics. Your child can use team or individual sports to combat the challenge of diabetes. Because diabetes can affect a child's body image, especially in terms of weight or feeling whole, mastering a sport is an excellent antidote. The child gains a sense of well-being and mastery. Liking one's body is important with or without diabetes. A good body image, developed through athletic involvement, can help the child want to take care of him or herself better. Athletics also help your child keep a good mood (exercise is an antidepressant) and lower blood glucose in the short and long run.

TEST TALK

Remember to be careful to take the judgment factor out of blood glucose testing. It is not a report card of your or your child's behavior. The word test implies judgment. Try using check instead. The results of checks must be considered neutral—only helpful information for problem solving and choosing future behaviors. Conversations around blood glucose results, particularly because they occur three or four times daily, must not be sources of anguish but rather routine sources of information for planning.

LETTING YOUR TEENAGER GROW UP

As time goes on, it is natural for your child to need to separate from you. Dr. LaGreca's research suggests that families who are positively involved with their kids during adolescence have children who follow diabetes management more closely. Children vary in intelligence, maturity, judgment, and decision-making ability. If you get anxious because they come home with new attitudes or behaviors, you will try to increase your control. This just leads to anger and resentment for both you and your children.

We need to understand that the major task of adolescents is to form an identity of their own, to become a

Mom: Did you check?
Son: I told you I hate when you ask me that. You know I haven't. I want you to remind me but the way you do seems like you are trying to catch me doing something wrong. **(positive assertion)**
Mom: You are right. **(nondefensive)** When you are done checking, why don't you come in and we can share some ideas about what is happening? **(assertive request)**
Son: (Later) It is 300.
Mom: Does it make sense to you? **(assertive questioning)**
Son: Yes. After school we all went for ice cream and everyone ordered hot fudge sundaes.
Mom: (Biting her lip to refrain from saying that from now on she will pick him up directly from school so he will not stop off with his friends). Is that what you felt like having or was it hard to order something different from your friends? **(assertive questioning)**
Son: (Shocked that she didn't lecture him) Actually, they all ordered two—had a pigout—and I was impressed with myself that I didn't go for the second one.
Mom: Sounds like you can make your own decisions and say no! **(positive reframing)** I am glad you are proud of yourself.
Son: Thanks. I'll be back, I'm going for a quick bike ride before dinner. **(independent problem solving)**

separate person, who still has close connections with family. It is the task of parents to assist your children in discovering what their personal beliefs and feelings are, separate from your own. Because you may have been told to expect adolescents to be moody and uncommunicative, you may allow communication to drop off between you and your kids. That—not adolescence—causes problems. Be a secure, steady presence in their lives.

With all that goes on during adolescence, diabetes care may get neglected. You must predict that physical growth spurts and fluctuating hormones can upset good diabetes control even if you do all the right things. Your child will feel frustration and a sense of personal failure when normal honest efforts are not rewarded with the usual outcomes, unless they are aware of this. At these times it is tempting for children to want to give up on control because no matter what they do, it still doesn't turn out right. Should they also have to deal with parents who might be critical or suspicious that it is from other causes? How do you want to impact your child's self-image concerns?

Diabetes can thread its way through all the issues of an adolescent's life—social acceptance, independence, invincibility, immediate gratification, spontaneity and decisions about driving safety, peer pressure and experimentation with drinking, drugs, sex, or smoking, and the future (occupation, having children, staying healthy). You need to empower your child to make informed decisions and choices, rather than operate out of fear or anger.

Susan, age 14, had done extremely well for the first 2 years she had diabetes. She had enjoyed the special attention given to diabetes, but she no longer received it. She was feeling upset about the diabetes because it was no longer new or special, and it had dawned on her that it was not going away. She was now trying to get attention based on ignoring her illness. Susan overheard her parents arguing about how expensive the blood testing strips were and expressing resentment about how ungrateful she seemed with all their efforts for her. She felt terrible that she had caused their fight and decided to stop testing out of anger, hurt, and not wanting to be a financial burden.

In a therapy session, the family listened to the story she was ready to share. They all lamented how difficult diabetes was and how they were burned out too. This honesty freed their compassion and quieted their anger at her poor diabetes care. They assured her that diabetes supplies fit in with their financial plans and that was their worry, not hers. Her job, having to take care of herself, was harder, and they were glad they could help with the finances.

With an adolescent, it is particularly difficult to determine what is diabetes related and what is a normal developmental issue. There are the normal times of irritability, impatience, striving for independence, and rebellion. These same responses can apply to having diabetes, and low blood sugar can appear as the same behaviors and need to be treated right away. Poor blood sugar control can contribute to moodiness, slow down maturation, and frustrate teens who are already superconscious of their bodies.

There are things you can do to help your teenager. Parents must exercise authority but with interest, compassion, and flexibility. Your child has special behavioral requirements—checking and recording blood sugar, carrying something to treat low blood sugar, wearing diabetes identification—that must be treated as normal, with normal reinforcements and consequences for doing or not doing them. Listen to your child's thoughts about what s/he has to do, and try to set up guidelines together—such as checking blood sugar before driving a car. It is up to your child, not you, to follow these guidelines. While you may share your values with your teenager, such as abstaining from alcohol or sex, your goal is to help them be safe in their choices. You could discuss your child having a designated watcher if s/he ever experiments with alcohol to avoid the low blood sugar that could result. You can point out the impact of alcohol on judgment and blood sugar (not to mention sexual matters) and the dangers of smoking in diabetes. Help teach your child's friends to recognize the symptoms and how to treat high and low blood sugars. Discuss sexual issues as you would anyway, with the specific additional burdens that having diabetes can bring (infections that can bring on high blood sugars and the importance of birth control and establishing normal blood sugars before getting pregnant to ensure the health of the baby). Encourage (and join) your child in healthy exercise or sports to regulate emotions, diabetes, and a healthy image for the changing body. Discuss good foot care. Enlist support from the medical team in helping your child internalize these good health practices as their own. Respect the resentment that comes from the additional worries that diabetes brings.

PREVENTING EATING DISORDERS IN YOUR TEENAGER

People with diabetes do have to have an unusual focus on food. In addition, our society is unnaturally focused on weight, dieting, and body image. Other pressures on your child can include the losses involved in diabetes itself, constant evaluation of self through blood sugar readings, the possible overinvolvement of a parent, biological depression from high blood sugars, and rapid weight changes. You can counteract these pressures with active grieving on diagnosis of diabetes, exercise for optimizing body image, positive family involvement, support groups, and preventive individual or family therapy.

Thanks to the new American Diabetes Association nutritional guidelines, restrictions and dieting are out and flexibility and lots of food choices—even fast foods and dessert—are in. Look at your own attitudes about food, eating, and body image, and realize that if you have distortions, you may pass them on to your children. The best place to start changing is to adopt some healthy eating practices and exercise goals for your own lifestyle. If you are concerned, get the help of your health care provider.

DIVORCED AND BLENDED STEPFAMILIES

There are special issues for any child who must fit into a divorced or blended-step family. The child probably will go through a period of anger, confusion, bitterness, or guilt. Adjustment takes time and families need patience and kindness and expectations of success. Be sure that the child with diabetes (and siblings) does not think s/he caused the divorce or that diabetes, in particular, did. Watch out for a diabetes crisis that may be a deliberate attempt to bring the natural parents back together

A new stepparent may be overwhelmed by diabetes. Other family members have to remember they had similar feelings in their own initial adjustment to diabetes. If you treat a child in a special way because of diabetes, that special attention will backfire into anger and rivalry with the other parent and siblings. It is tough for a child to handle diabetes and divorce. You can prepare yourself and your children for these crises by reading books that predict and help solve the issues that will come up for the new family.

There is grieving for the old family but there is potential for important relationships in the new family. Parents need to speak to each other often and find agreement on parenting principles. Be quick to forgive things that may have been done or said in the adjustment period, for example a stepdaughter putting the new stepmother down in front of the other children. Parents must do a lot to reinforce each other because these difficult times will probably not include much appreciation by the children. (That is true for parenting, in general.) Be consistent, appreciate your partner and yourself.

Peter was diagnosed with diabetes at age 6, and his parents divorced when he was 8. He and his mother were very close and did lots of special things together. Even at 8, Peter knew what being the "man of the house" meant. When his mother, Barbara, began to date Walter a year later, he was edgy but pleased in general to have a man paying special attention to him. Peter and his mom still had their special times and secrets. And then it hit Peter drastically. He now had to share his best friend, his mother, and worse, she would no longer keep his secrets. Walter seemed to know everything. Why did his mother need another man to take care of her? In Peter's mind, he had already been abandoned by his father who did not see him regularly, and now he was losing his mother, too. It was worse when Walter and his mother married. She had never bossed him around, but now she let this man rule over him. And it was spreading to telling him what to do with his diabetes, too.

Everyone had adjustments to make, which would take time, listening, and acceptance by the parents of Peter's feelings. He had to accept the loss of his exclusive best friend, recognize that the harshness demonstrated by his new stepfather was partly attributable to jealousy of the special mother-son closeness, and accept the new but necessary (and actually relieving) boundaries of parents being in charge. Peter was going to gain a loving stepfather, and he was going to be able to focus on growing up rather than taking care of his mom.

If the stepparent has diabetes, these guidelines still count and diabetes care must come first. The children may be fearful, disinterested, or not understand your diabetes in the beginning, just as they are not sure about you replacing their other parent. Be careful not to turn the disappointments you experience back on the family or yourself or your diabetes. Don't put energy into feeling injured, put it into trying again. Read books to see what is normal, and keep talking to your partner. Your good relationship will be the anchor for making the family work. It will improve with time if you expect some hard times and don't hold grudges along the way.

SINGLE PARENTS

Single parents have their own set of challenges. They must enlist others—friends, their own parents, other parents of children with diabetes, and baby-sitters. Overinvolvement and burnout are risks when you are the only one doing the parenting. The financial strains of raising a family alone are magnified by the additional costs of diabetes care and having to leave work in an emergency. More than ever, the single parent must create a network that really offers support and relief. You'll need to take an adult break for yourself for perspective, relief, and some fun. You may need to get over a fear of imposing on others to get it. You are not imposing when your great kid, who happens to have diabetes, spends time with another family or relative. They are getting the joys of your child and the pleasure of learning to do something difficult. They are also lending support to a friend. Don't limit other people's rewards because your false pride says you must do it all on your own.

CHILDREN LEAVING HOME

Eventually your child will go off to college or to work and live independently. You may find this an especially emotional time, and your children may be disturbed about leaving you, too. All of you must do your best to build full lives and not be preoccupied with each other. Independence is healthy—it's what you've all been working toward. Enjoy yours, too.

Your children with diabetes may have trouble separating or may feel overjoyed at the opportunity. Likewise, you may have ambivalence about cutting the cord. Going away means your child will be making decisions (despite all the phone calls home) on many things: getting up on time, doing laundry, managing money and meals, figuring out priorities and getting school and social tasks completed, study skills, time management, getting enough sleep, solving problems, and handling illnesses. Hard enough. Throw diabetes in. This makes letting go even harder. For both of you. You'll worry about your child running out of diabetes supplies, ordering them, handling sick-day rules, handling low blood glucose—who will know and know how to help—and figuring out what to eat. (By now your children have internalized your "voice of reason.")

It may help you both to rehearse some of these situations ahead of time. It also means keeping the link, being supportive, and expecting success—don't let anxiety run the show. Enlist the help of your health professionals to go over the specifics of diabetes care in relation to alcohol, drugs, sexual activity, peer pressure, foot care, etc. Encourage your child to develop a good relationship with health care providers all through life and help him or her find a new health team in the vicinity. Maybe you can role play telling new friends about diabetes.

Young people leaving home should be able to talk to you without undermining their independence. The trick is to give help when it is asked for and reinforce their successes. It may be natural to want to call more and nag and question. Neither one of you will feel good if you do that.

WHEN YOUR CHILD GETS MARRIED

Figuring out a way to hand off the torch to a well-meaning partner of your child with diabetes can be difficult. You can hope and expect that the values you put into your child's head about health and family will take root in this new relationship. They need to separate from you, to make their own unit together. Later, they will most likely include you in their lives (and not just because they need money).

Be patient and understanding of this normal developmental process with steady but nonintrusive interest in both of them, and it will most likely pay off. Being an ally and supporter, not competitor or critic, is a satisfying role to play. Refer them to chapter 7 on couples.

Couples

In every marriage or similar relationship, partners look for a chance to bond, highlighting emotional and physical connection.

Partners come into a marriage with explicit but perhaps unknown expectations of what a marriage is and what each wants from the other. These revelations come out over time, satisfying or shocking the individuals involved but nonetheless providing an opportunity for growth and change. The major goal of a good marriage is to finish growing up. We can get past the childhood scars and gender hurdles that must be crossed, form an individual identity that fits flexibly within the marital relationship, and create a satisfying relationship built on love and respect.

After a fight with her husband, Sue, who has diabetes, goes into the kitchen and loudly bangs the cabinet doors. Sue mutters to herself about how mad she is at her husband, Paul. She yells out, "Hope you know exactly where you are driving me!"

It sounds like emotional blackmail, the unfortunate option we sometimes take when another person does not respond the way we want. It is tempting to regain power by making the other feel guilty or responsible for our actions, as in this case. At other times, it is enticing to threaten to take away our love or approval when we don't get our way.

It is up to you not to get caught in the web. This is the way to save you both. The *winner* is the first person to understand or find the source of the problem. Blackmail is hazardous for everyone's health. In this situation, the good news is that Sue is announcing her planned reaction, letting her husband know she is helpless and upset. This is healthier because she is not choosing to sneak food in response to feeling badly.

The situation has potential for a positive outcome. Her husband can hear her message and decide to feel guilty or angry and respond in the same way, making the situation worse for both of them. The alternative is for him to take 5 deep breaths and decide to hear her cry for help, behind what sounds like blame. Paul can come into the kitchen, or if he hasn't taken enough deep breaths and is still furious, he can yell from the other room.

"I know you are upset with me. Give me some time to think about what you have said. Why punish **yourself** by eating, getting high blood sugars, and feeling guilty? If you really want to get back at me, only me, hide the TV remote control."

If this attempt at recognizing her feelings, demonstrating caring, and distraction through humor doesn't work to help Sue, at least it cuts out the unnecessary self-blaming that could follow for her husband. One wounded person at a time is enough.

Most situations are not so simple that you have only one emotional response. Unfortunately we often react to the feeling that comes first. It is important to recognize what these feelings are, so that your response and then the interactions between you two are not based on peripheral matters, but are about the real issue. The real issues are having a nice day, safeguarding your partner's health, maintaining your own health, and making sure your marriage contract is healthy—by the way you speak to each other and how you love and help each other.

Without self-awareness, you can go on to say things that will have a harmful effect on all those aspects of your life and your partner's life. The choice is yours. If you do express yourself, you may be satisfied, but you will likely have to learn to tolerate that s/he may be upset with you.

Remember that in communication each person is both a sender and a receiver. The more skills you use to decipher incoming messages and then send your own messages, the smoother your relationship and diabetes care will go.

When one partner has diabetes, there can be many changes in your life, all of which are difficult at first. The challenges may cover the range of dealing with a partner's denial of diabetes, mealtime conflicts, watching out for low blood glucose, fighting over high blood glucose, dealing with the financial extras, fearing complications, and difficult feelings such as fear, anger, or disappointment. Those real feelings occur, but living with diabetes can provide opportunities for focusing on living one day at a time, healthy eating, exercising regularly, and living on a higher spiritual plane that emphasizes enjoying each other and what you have. Most people live in a take-it-

Your partner with diabetes, with whom you fought earlier in the morning, calls you when s/he arrives at work. S/he says in an angry voice, "My blood sugar is up. I can't have you yelling at me before I go to work. You are ruining my health." You say:

1. I guess I mess up everything. (guilt)
2. You blame everyone else for what you don't take care of. (accuracy and anger)
3. I am glad you called. **(positive reframing)** I am sure you are worried. It must be a terrible feeling to think that other people, not you, are in control of your blood sugars. Would you like me to help you look at this differently? **(assertive empathy/request)**
4. You are right, the best time to talk is not right before work. **(nondefensive)** We need to make times to discuss the issues annoying us. **(assertive request).** Have a good day. I am going to have a great one.

Answer evaluation

1. Guilt just puts you down and makes you feel bad about yourself. It usually aggravates the other person, although it can often keep him quiet for a while. It does distract you both from the important issue.
2. This may be a good insight, very accurate, in fact, but delivered in this way and at this time, it is a bit aggressive. Your partner is at work and cannot really hear it or respond to it. You don't get a good reputation for sensitivity, either.
3. This goes right for the empathy connection. It is nicely nondefensive and focuses on the positive and on solving the problem.
4. This is good, too. It is looking for agreement on the issues that you can both accept. It confirms the need for time to be set aside to talk about it. Both are part of having a good marriage.

for-granted state or comfort zone and can miss opportunities to value what is important now. The requirements of diabetes, even healthy check-ups, can be a catalyst to get you moving into this positive consciousness of enjoying life now. Remember, life is not a dress rehearsal.

A GUIDE FOR PARTNERS

Here are some good ideas for all couples (even those who don't have a chronic illness in the family). (See Laura Epstein Rosen and Xavier Francisco Amador's book, *When Someone You Love is Depressed: How to Help Your Loved One Without Losing Yourself.*)

1. Talk out the issues.

2. Don't neglect your needs or feelings. Neither of you should be ashamed about feeling anger and resentment at diabetes because those feelings are natural when living with chronic illness. There is often relief when you can voice what you are worried or annoyed about for both you and your partner. Don't get mired down in guilt and responsibility.

3. Do give support. This can come in the form of listening and positive coaching as well as learning as much as you can about diabetes—including how to test blood sugars, give glucagon injections, recognize and help treat low blood glucose reactions, help with meal plans, and trying to enjoy exercise. All this participation makes you healthier, too. People are more likely to lower their health risk factors if their spouses are doing it, too.

4. Help the person with diabetes get good ongoing and preventive help, in addition to your help. There are lots of health care professionals who can lighten the load for both of you. A support team can help keep problems from getting out of hand. If your partner doesn't want to ask for help, make sure you get some help to figure out how to handle the situation and your feelings and interactions. You are only in control of what *you* do differently, not your partner.

5. Identify and solve problems as they come up. Substance abuse or depression in one partner can trigger increased fighting and sexual or marital difficulties. Those are not normal states, even if couples get used to them. Resentment, loneliness, or sadness are signals of trouble and must be heeded. In fact, welcome them as caution signs that one or both of you is probably in emotional trouble. Not taking care of emotional problems leads to problems in any marriage and can also lead to physical problems of diabetes. It takes two to make problems, and two to fix them. Be honest with each other and determined to find new, more harmonious ways of living together. Get help from qualified mental health professionals.

6. Understand that your partner's rejection of your help is usually about him or her, not the rejection of you as a person. If your partner spurns your interest in diabetes, it can mean any of a number of things. Perhaps the rejection is a symptom of depression and helplessness that s/he feels and may be unable to identify. It might be a bad mood, resulting from poor diabetic control. It could be that, to your partner, needing help means feeling inferior, inadequate, or unable to take care of him or herself. Do not assume your partner does not need help just because s/he is refusing your interest. Try not to waste energy feeling hurt because your partner is not responding in the way you want. Figure out new ways to get your message across and take care of yourself. Spend time on the skills involved in different communication styles discussed later in this chapter.

7. Remind your partner that diabetes is a joint issue, "ours" just like sex and money.

8. Highlight normalcy, wellness, and positive experiences together. Diabetes is not who you are or who the couple is. It needs to be respected but kept in perspective. To be alive and rich, a marriage needs fun, positive surprises, and occasional returns to how it was at the beginning—going out of your way to think of your partner first. Live one day at a time, maximizing all the pleasures that you have at the moment.

DIFFERENT COPING STYLES OF PARTNERS

As we focus on how individuals cope with diabetes, it is important to consider the coping style of the partner without diabetes, too. You may neglect your own well-being because you are preoccupied with your partner. You may unconsciously hide your own meaningful issues behind your partner's illness. Good intentions aside, reacting to your partner's diabetes with overwhelming anxiety can make your partner feel guilty about causing you pain. During a husband's transition into retirement, for example, he may begin to constantly ask his wife, "How are you feeling? Why aren't you smiling?"—driving them both crazy. His feelings about his own retirement, changing roles, or aging have been denied, and he may become preoccupied with controlling his wife's health instead. If what is really going on is recognized, then the right person gets help, and they both avoid creating new problems.

Coping style differences may work to your benefit. For example, if your partner is more disciplined or compulsive, s/he can help by reminding you about testing, when to eat, or to bring a snack. In some cases, your partner's coping style may be irritating. For instance a compulsive worrier may seem to be always watching you, treating you as a sick person, or asking the same questions repeatedly. This could undermine your self-confidence or provoke rebellion, much the same way an adolescent responds to an overbearing parent. Quality of life—being healthy, mutually satisfied, and communicating well—is essential to both of you in the marriage. See how your coping styles can complement each other.

MARRIAGE TASKS

Dr. Ruth Wallerstein, the author of *Good Marriage*, wrote the book because of her concern that one in two marriages ends in divorce and that one in three children live in a divorced home. She became very interested in identifying the tasks and goals of marriage and providing some insight on the prevention of breakups.

Her breakdown of these tasks is similar to the issues we have already discussed in having a healthy family (see chapter 5). Once again, these are the same issues

DR. WALLERSTEIN'S TASKS OF MARRIAGE ARE:

- separating from the parents to join in the new relationship
- maintaining togetherness and separateness in the marriage
- confronting the challenges of life—including children and health—with an enhanced relationship
- building a safe place for conflict, good sex, laughter, and nurturance
- creating a place to store past and present memories

and strategies that help you and your partner take care of your diabetes.

THE IN-LAWS

Parents naturally wonder if anyone will consider their children's needs with as much concern and knowledge as they did. Before the parents hand over the baton, there may be double soul searching to make sure this new daughter or son-in-law will be a positive part of the diabetes challenges as well. Likewise the parents may feel jealousy, though pleasure, that the son- or daughter-in-law is more successfully involved than they were.

People with a chronic illness need their supportive loved ones from the past and the present to be capable and close by. It is the manner of how to stay involved that needs careful attention.

To avoid the change in status from in-law to outlaw, all parties need to remain open, tolerant of roles changing, and very forgiving.

The parents of the child who marries someone with diabetes may have another set of feelings. They may be worried about what diabetes will mean for their adult child. Their first reaction may not be to support but to fear and challenge, concerned that their child will be emotionally and financially burdened.

Once your parents know your fiancé and have information about the disease, their skepticism is more often than not supplanted with loving concern. They may be educated by the person with diabetes, professionals on the medical team, or by reading current diabetes literature. They should grow to respect the maturity and depth of your choice, even when things might not be easy for you.

COMBINING FREEDOM AND HEALTHY DEPENDENCE

In the beginning couples often exhaust themselves by expecting each other to agree and validate each other 100% of the time as part of the "we" process. Eventually you need to move to a point of not losing your individual selves (the "I") but live it in the context of "we," acknowledging the value of both parties at the same time, even with conflict. Without this ability to differentiate, Dr. David Schnarch, author of *Passionate Marriage*, suggests that couples will find themselves controlling each other, overriding personal needs for the sake of the other, or receding into the background. This emotional growth pattern pertains to issues of sex and decisions about finances and childrearing, as well as health issues.

In a new marriage, creating a new identity of "we" without forgetting about "I" is a big challenge. In this second task of marriage, diabetes needs to be important to both people. Neither one of you should get off track in taking care of your own health for the sake of the other person and the marriage.

Communicating what you expect and need, nurturing each other, and fighting fair can preserve the "I" priority and create a healthy "we."

People with type 1 or type 2 diabetes must look at the effect that diabetes has on their relationships with their spouse and children. Taking care of yourself, to prevent depression and the risk of poor health, aids marital adjustment. A healthy marriage, in turn, produces healthier relationships with your children. The themes and stresses in a marriage change with your, your partner's, and your children's life cycles. Be aware of other stresses on your marriage so you can cope with them and keep them from derailing your diabetes care.

PREGNANCY

Pregnancy is a critical and life-changing event for any woman. It involves physical and emotional changes such as new roles, a fluctuating body image, and new worries. The added demands of the pregnancy regimen for a woman with diabetes, focusing on tight blood glucose control for the health of the baby, magnifies her stress.

We know that tight diabetes control before becoming pregnant is equally important for the developing fetus. Sometimes the pregnancy is the first time the woman really pays attention to herself. Where there are difficulties in adherence or in the marriage prior to the pregnancy, this can be a good time for crisis intervention counseling, helping the woman to do her best in having a successful pregnancy, a better attitude for long-lasting health care, and a stronger marriage.

WHEN THE PERSON WITH DIABETES HAS A CHILD WITH DIABETES

Jim, who had had diabetes for 25 years, appeared to handle his son's diagnosis of diabetes very well. Two months later, he was rushed to the hospital, thinking he was having a heart attack. It turned out that he was fine physically, but the stress from guilt and fear had taken over his body. Life was not fair to him, but it devastated him that now it was not fair to his son either.

A lot of soul searching and suffering went on for him. When he looked at his son with all the love and affection he had always felt for him, could he wish even for a second that he had not had him? When he thought about how much plea-

sure and happiness he had in his own life, and much of it from his son, could he not hope that his son would grow up happy with his diabetes and look forward to creating his own family?

With this opportunity to continue his own grieving, he accepted his son's diagnosis and resolved to upgrade his own care. He was clearly a model for his son now, and he wanted to remove, as much as possible, the shame or discomfort about his own diabetes. He did not want to give his son bitterness or sadness. Together they were going to have to turn this thing around and focus on the special bond that would bring them even closer. They were going to think of this as an opportunity to operate as their own special 24-hour support group, helping each other with good habits and good decisions and a sense of pride.

RAISING CHILDREN

Raising children often gets in the way of good diabetes habits. I think the airlines are right when they tell passengers that in case of an emergency, they should put the oxygen masks over their own faces before taking care of their children. At first, that information seems selfish. Looking closer, it becomes obvious that you would not be of any help to your child if you did not take care of yourself first. So it goes in diabetes.

EFFECT OF PARENTS' DIABETES ON CHILDREN

Children usually feel anxiety about their parents' vulnerability. Be careful not to put undue responsibility, pressure, or guilt on the children about your daily or long-term health. "Thanks, kids, for your support in taking bike rides with me. I take care of myself, but it pleases me that you help." You would be better off not going to their favorite restaurant if you have been having trouble lately eating more than you wanted to in those places. "Thanks, kids, for being such good sports, even though I know it is disappointing to you to give up your favorite restaurant for a while." This is a nice message of appreciation rather than a burden the children must accept.

Prioritizing your health is not harmful to anyone else's health. If anything, it sets a good example for your family members to follow in their own lives, whether it is eating well, exercising, or thinking of their own needs in the context of caring about others, too.

Your child can have subtle worries about the present (low blood glucose and many doctor appointments) and the future (how long will my parent be there for me? Will I get diabetes, too?) Again, it is important that you have your own healthy view of life with a chronic disease—you are careful about taking care of yourself and expect to stay healthy—so that is the message relayed to your child.

Children can feel inhibited about imposing and having their needs met when they view you as sick. They can feel guilty when you have low blood glucose episodes, feeling that they may have caused it. They can be reluctant at times to go through the normal adolescent rebellion—the task of separating from the family—feeling afraid that they will hurt their already vulnerable parent. It sounds funny to say, but being free to be angry at your parents is a rite of passage.

HELP EACH OTHER KEEP PERSPECTIVE

Miranda, a 35-year-old woman with type 1 diabetes was aware that she would refuse her daughter's requests to drive her places by saying that she did not feel well rather than just saying, "No, get another ride this time." She was afraid of her child's disappointment and anger being turned on her, and she avoided the conflict of having to say no. She knew her daughter would not argue with her if she were sick. In this case, diabetes was used, unnecessarily, as a disability and a way to avoid honest problem solving. Members in the family unnecessarily felt secondary to the diabetes. Diabetes was center stage in a dysfunctional way. Miranda's behavior may look selfish and manipulative, but in therapy, she revealed situations that made her behavior seem to be an extension of what she had learned as a kid.

Miranda remembered frequent incidences where family members had used her diabetes to get out of things, too. Her older brother would tell the people at work he could not work on Saturdays because he had to watch his kid sister with diabetes. Sometimes her parents would use her diabetes as an excuse to get out of invitations. It had seemed natural for her to get out of doing things she was afraid to try as a child, too, because of her diabetes. So here she was, doing what comes naturally, as an adult. She could see how detrimental this was for her and certainly for her daughter. She was determined not to hurt her child and knew she needed to do something different now.

In therapy, Miranda learned and practiced the skills in compassionate no-saying. She began to understand that she did not have to say yes, even if she felt fine! She thought about how all of her family had experienced anxiety in social situations and had used her illness to avoid the reality of their own personal fears. She began a process of recognizing her own anxieties and tried to use her intellect to get rid of them. Miranda began to see herself as hardy and healthy and spread that idea to her daughter, too. They laughed together as a family that she was becoming selfish and healthy, saying no to their requests.

Her daughter came into therapy and learned to be more open and to confront her mother on issues that disturbed her. Now when her mother said no to her, she could voice her objections, challenge her, and even walk away angry. If she found later that her mother's blood sugars were elevated, she would know clearly that she was not the cause. The father learned to stop saying, "Don't bother your mother, she doesn't feel well." The father also had not bothered the mother because she didn't feel well, and their relationship had been suffering, too. He joined them in learning to recognize and express his needs as well.

SEX

Good sexual relations are important for any marriage. Sex is communication, intimacy, creativity, habit, physical expression, and satisfaction. Sex comes through in two parts: desire and actual physical connection. Out of control blood glucose can bring mood changes that can alter or inhibit sexual interest for both men and women. Long-term poorly controlled blood glucose and acute low blood glucose can effect temporary or permanent performance problems in men. For women, poorly controlled blood glucose can lead to yeast infections, a loss of nerve sensation, poor body image, self-consciousness, and actual physical discomfort from decreased vaginal lubrication—all of which inhibit sexual enjoyment, but most of which can be anticipated and controlled.

Don't misinterpret a temporary lack of drive or ability as permanent or even diabetes related. It may just be a part of the normal stresses of living. Most people without diabetes experience changing sexual drives or an inability to achieve or maintain an erection or achieve orgasm for some period through the course of their lives.

A satisfying sex life is one of the reasons that good blood glucose control is in the interest of more than the person with diabetes. Even if there are temporary or permanent problems, diabetes should not be in the way, permanently, of a satisfying sexual life to both partners. Getting professional help can tackle any preexisting marital or sexual problems in addition to concerns with the current physical functioning. Lovemaking, which needs to be sustained in any marriage, is much more than performance or intercourse. A sexual relationship is accomplished with communication, playfulness, and laughter, not necessarily an end point of intercourse. Dr. Schnarch suggests patients try "hugging till relaxed" as a nonsexual basis for connecting emotionally. Even when there are no emotional or physical problems, talking about sex can be difficult. A good time to start is when all is going well. Good communication habits established by talking over what is significant or pleasurable to you is a reliable place to begin. It involves overcoming the possible embarrassment or concerns that so many people worry about when discussing anything, let alone sex. Other communication fears include concern that it means giving up spontaneity and risking rejection or causing conflict. It is so easy to forget that conversation more often leads to intimacy, safety, and satisfaction.

Discussing your sex life with your health professionals is also important. Your medical team should be able to be direct and persistent with you and your partner to keep you from avoiding identifying a problem. Depression itself may cause changes in sexual interest or functioning, but some medications for treatment of depression may also lead to changes in desire or lubrication for women, libido or performance for men and difficulty reaching orgasm for both. Patients who won't discuss these issues are left on their own, and they may discontinue, in frustration, the antidepressants or hypertension medications, which they assume are causing sexual problems. Don't make changes without consulting your doctor, who can make decisions with you about lowering doses, taking "drug holidays" (stopping for a few weekend days), or switching to medications that don't have those side effects.

Men should not expect to have a loss or change in their sexual functioning. If there is a change in your ability to have and maintain an erection, get information about the temporary or permanent nature of impotency. If the change is permanent, you must grieve over the loss and changes, and so must your partner. Your feelings of pride must be respected but cannot take over the need for communication between partners. A professional third party can help with information and communication suggestions. The understandable grief must not get stuck in anger or sadness. Both partners' sexual needs can be addressed over time. Individual needs, including differences must be taken into consideration. For example, Ann Landers did a study suggesting that women preferred foreplay over intercourse. What you expect or need from your sexual relationship will change over your lifetime. Don't limit it unnecessarily.

If there are changes, a couple must begin to talk to each other. For example, a woman who sees that her husband is avoiding sexual contact may incorrectly assume it is about her and become depressed or suspicious. It would be much more helpful to her to know that he is avoiding contact because of his concern over not being able to maintain erections. Together they could then work on achieving tighter blood glucose control for him and change the sexual timing or stimulation in their encounters. They should speak to their doctor about assessing the problem—such as hormonal evaluations or duplex Doppler ultrasound for blood flow within the penis—and whether to try hormonal supplements, vacuum therapy, injections, or the new oral drug for impotence. If there is an irreversible problem, they could keep their sex life strong through alternative means—manual emphases, sexual aids, surgical implants, or just plain touch. Let me underscore what we have talked about all along. Become knowledgeable about the facts and the feelings and when in doubt, talk to each other and to your health care team.

FINANCIAL ISSUES

It may surprise you to know that finances are perhaps the most stressful and least talked about issue between couples. People feel very private about money issues. Most of us have our own idiosyncrasies. Diabetes does put a financial drain on the family budget. No way around it. Even though most families are covered by insurance, there are still large out-of-pocket costs that clearly impact on financial decisions being made within a home. (See chapter 6.)

Financial considerations can bring a vast array of feelings for you with diabetes and your partner. You may have your own resentment or guilt about spending the money, taking it away from other areas you would rather be spending on for yourself or the family. Your partner, too, may have reasonable feelings of resentment and then guilt for having those feelings, too. S/he may feel entitled to demand good blood glucose control from you because s/he gives up other things for contributing to the diabetes budget. You may resent this, feeling it is an attempt at controlling you or feeling that it is your diabetes. All feelings are okay. The problem is the extreme action of self-destructive thinking: "Never mind, I will take nothing and owe you nothing and therefore you can't tell me about my diabetes." You and your partner are always entitled to share your needs and feelings but you need a common goal.

I have observed that patients who could afford their medicines, at times so resented the need for them and the high prices that they stopped taking them in silent protest. This backfires when anxiety and depression interfere with good self-care. Patients become too anxious to exercise, monitor, or eat well, and they attempt to alleviate their bad feelings by eating more.

People who truly cannot afford medications have to figure out ways to get them with the help of doctors or public agencies. Other people may be able to pay but feel they cannot afford things. Sometimes this is accurate. The truth about their financial ability to pay is an emotional issue, with the patient questioning himself as a priority in the family budget, looking for a way to hide from the demands of diabetes, or making excuses to express anger or denial of just how important self-care is.

It is dangerous to be shortsighted about spending the amount of money that it takes to stay healthy through the years. Good health is central to being a satisfying partner and parent, including being happy, healthy, and able to work. Diabetes is not fair to any of you. However, if you do not value or take care of yourself, that is more unfair. No matter how personal the money issue feels, it must be discussed.

No career moves can be made without thinking about getting adequate health insurance, life insurance, earning enough money for medical expenses, or which job has the best health care plan with the right specialists on their lists. Couples have to learn to ask the right questions of HMOs.

In the past, and perhaps still in the present, changing jobs is a challenge because of limited coverage for preexisting illnesses. One patient had trouble getting hired because insurance for her kidney transplant maintenance would be very expensive for the firms she was applying to. Legally, of course, they could not discriminate and avoid hiring her for that reason. The reality was something different. Hopefully, things are changing for the better on these issues.

Besides the costs of medicines, supplies, and diabetes education, there is the expense of going to the many specialists who are involved in preventing complications. These specialists add to the expense of health care maintenance: foot doctors (podiatrists), dentists, ophthalmologists, nurse educators, dietitians, psychologists, and exercise specialists, and perhaps later, neurologists, cardiologists, or nephrologists. There are laws being proposed to cover prevention and education services for people with diabetes, because these are the most effective treatments.

EXPECTATIONS OF THE PARTNER WITHOUT DIABETES

We have to distinguish between caring about the person and being upset with the behaviors of that person. Either partner may be concerned when the other one is not thoughtful or helpful about health issues or efforts. Your partner expects you to follow your diabetes plan. You show your efforts through discussion with your partner periodically about your goals, what helps, what is a disappointment, what you hope for, and by going together to regular visits to the health care team.

You and your partner can find additional help. Attend support groups such as weight watchers, overeaters anonymous, or 12-step programs for eating or alcohol problems. Go to exercise programs, gyms, or individual physical trainers. Seek referrals to professionals when evaluation and medication might help with anxiety, depression, or specific weight loss. All of these take money and time. Each takes effort—and appreciation of that effort, too.

MAKING IT WORK

Part of being a good partner is being able to step back from nagging or criticism—ineffective anyway—to determine what is really going on. There may, in fact, be underlying depression, anxiety, or perhaps a preexisting compulsive eating disorder. Helping your spouse get to the appropriate health professional will make all of the difference in the world to successful diabetes management and a healthy person and marriage. People often resist getting help, whether it is in the form of seeing specialists or taking the medicines they prescribe. Conversations about this resistance have to include hearing the reasons and then presenting loving challenges to grow.

Getting help can mean many things. Giving up the relative comfort of procrastination and actually facing a problem causes anxiety. It can mean helplessness, inferiority, or a loss of pride; a move away from rugged individualism (particularly for men); giving up control; and resentment for feeling indebted. These feelings are powerful. Often patients begin by telling me they don't want the crutch of prescribed antidepressant medication, and then wince when they realize how they already lean on glasses of wine, food, and over-the-counter pills to cope with stress.

Deana, who was obese for most of her adult life, was diagnosed with diabetes at age 45. Not surprisingly, she continued to be overweight. Her husband got furious that now she had a medical reason to lose weight, but she could not do it. He was disturbed by what he called her "weak will" and uncaring attitude about herself or him. He grew more angry with her every day.

Her medical team determined that she had a compulsive eating disorder, which if left untreated, would leave her diabetes in shambles. A referral was made to a psychiatrist, specializing in psychopharmacology. She started medications, because Deana's eating habits were partly a response to biological deficits. With a combination of medications normally used for treating anxiety and depression, Deana actually experienced fewer food cravings. Once she could have some control over her compulsion to eat, she found herself more open to learning about how to make healthy food choices. For the first time, feeling in control of her cravings, she had a sense that she might even be able to control diabetes.

In sessions with her psychologist and nurse practitioner, she worked alone and with her husband to restore her self-image, shattered by many years of shame. Judgmental attitudes from physicians, society, herself, and family members who had scolded her for poor self-control contributed to this shame. Understanding the issues in a totally new light, her husband became an ally rather than an adversary. Both realized they had misread her irritability, fatigue, impatience, and compulsive eating as character issues rather than as symptoms of depression. They had not understood the symptoms as biological and psychological problems.

Without efforts to communicate, the partner without diabetes can become lost in resentment and frustration, feeling s/he is living with someone who does not seem to care about either one of them. It is human nature to find it difficult to love someone who does not seem to act lovingly to him or herself. Most people find it attractive in a person, even sexy, to see someone they love do healthy things. (Exercise produces something real: endorphin release, the body's natural high or pain killer.) You don't want to lose this whole area of closeness and intimacy. Staying distant or disinterested in yourself or your partner damages more than your health. It is the process of trying to stay healthy that fosters love and bonding and intimacy.

Unfortunately we cut each other off all the time, without intending to. Your partner may say she is afraid to go to the doctor. You say, "That is foolish. There is nothing to worry about." Or, you may say to your partner that it is your fault that he doesn't exercise, and you feel guilty. Your partner responds with "That's silly. It's my problem." You can hear the positive intention of the replies, but they actually dismiss the other person's feelings. You are relegated to feeling what you should feel rather than what you actually do feel. A simple "Tell me more. I would like to understand your feelings. Why are you are saying that?" would be setting the tone for mutual respect and support.

Sue and Dave have been married for 25 years. They argued, in the beginning, about his nonadherence to his diabetes plan. Almost every meal included a fight over the way the food was fixed or how much Dave ate. The arguments seemed to make the behaviors worse. No surprise. Adults can act out the same rebellion to their spouses that adolescents do with their parents.

Dave was angry with himself that he was not able to be effective with his diabetes. He was furious that his wife was angry at him for not following through. Sue seemed to constantly disapprove of him, but he wasn't seeing the whole picture. When Dave's blood sugars were high, he would be irritable and sluggish, fall asleep on the couch, avoid sexual contact, and sleep late the next day. He was not able to sustain the couple connection through affection, conversation, or physical communication. Sue was also frustrated with herself that she could not help him. Yet, he seemed to blame her for not doing enough to help him. She was already feeling guilty, and he seemed to throw more on top of her. Their marriage had moved from a passionately angry place to a listless, depressed, disappointed state.

In general, they needed to talk to each other. Dave was too lonely in his diabetes and blamed diabetes for causing all their fights and for keeping them distant from each other. Each needed to understand the other's feelings.

They talked about guidelines for finding intimacy without becoming overinvolved or trying to control each other. All they needed at first was to be able to hear each other and listen. Next, simple acknowledgment that each had heard would suffice. This meant not overreacting, not fixing, not needing success from the other person.

OVERINVOLVED

Sue: You ate so much cake at dinner. You always eat too much, get high blood sugars, and are no fun. All you do is fall asleep watching the TV.
Dave: I fall asleep because it is boring to hear you nag and complain or threaten through the whole dinner.

HEALTHY DETACHMENT

Sue: (Putting her hand lovingly on Dave's arm before they go out for dinner.) I want to tell you what my expectations are without turning you off. We both know you choose, of course, to do whatever you like. Here is what I am hoping for. I am looking forward to a sensual evening during and after dinner. I hope to have a special dessert for you when we get home. I hope you will keep your blood sugars normal so that you can stay up for it (I mean not fall asleep) and enjoy it.
Dave: (Breathe in, breathe out.) I am having a big flash of resentment. On the other hand, I guess I am also glad you are trying something new, being more positive. I like this conversation when you take care of yourself by telling me your feelings and expectations, rather than what I should do. (He is beginning to soften and be receptive.) I want to make good choices. It is very hard for me when we go out for dinner. I find this helpful. It feels good to anticipate pleasures and problems. Why don't you move the bread basket after we each take a piece?

They needed to "mind their own business" and yet be interested in, but not take over, each other's domains.

This point of "healthy detachment" included sharing needs and being involved with the other person. That does not mean you cannot have feelings about what your partner does. You can tell *your* feelings and needs about a situation, not what the other person needs to do.

Of course this sounds stilted. Dave and his wife are trying on some new behaviors. But stilted beats guilted.

THE POWER OF INTERACTIONS

We affect each other. When the mood is set right, conversation can lead to some *problem solving* about the difficulty of eating out. Even more important, it leads to intimacy. Relationships are powerful in helping us to feel good about ourselves and helping us move closer to our goals.

There are things you may want your partner to know how to do such as test your blood glucose, recognize your hypoglycemia, and help you treat it, and give glucagon injections. Some people want their spouses to read about diabetes and attend classes or learn to cook and eat in healthy ways. Some want their partners to go with them to doctors' appointments and sometimes go instead of them! People who seem to want to do everything on their own may be repeating (or rebelling against) learned patterns of relationships. Or perhaps they don't want to be watched and criticized, found out, or put too much worry on the other person. This is probably like the adolescent who does better with support, but resists it all along the way. The power of couples working together, helping each other, can strengthen a marriage and help with diabetes care.

LOW BLOOD GLUCOSE

Agree on a plan in advance of ways to prevent and treat low blood glucose. Resistance to getting help is often part of the low blood glucose reaction. Unfortunately, partners sometimes take this rejection of help at the time of the low blood glucose as the way the partner really feels.

My experience over the years suggests that we must not remember the words or attitudes spewed out during what I call the low blood sugar precipice—the period of time, as the blood glucose is dropping, characterized by unpleasantly memorable mood changes.

John is 35 years old. He is intelligent, conscientious, meticulous, and a delightful person. He was diagnosed at 30 and the doctors started out controlling his diabetes without insulin. It was determined quickly that his body needed insulin, despite all his efforts at eating and exercising well. He was tremendously disappointed. John was determined that he, and not the medication, was going to control his diabetes. He tried to eat as little as he could and compulsively exercised after every meal so that he, not the insulin, brought the blood sugar down. He would often not take a snack before bedtime, even if he might go low; he preferred being low to possibly waking up with a high blood sugar. He would feel a sense of helplessness before bedtime, knowing that he could not impact his blood sugars during sleep. In short, John did not like depending on insulin.

John was a model patient in terms of his goals—normal blood glucose levels—but not really ideal in the way he was going about getting there. He was using undue deprivation, discipline, and anxiety. Approximately four times a month for the last several months, Sara could not wake John up in the mornings before work. Because she was afraid to learn to give glucagon injections and the responsibility it entailed, her only recourse was to call the ambulance for help. While his blood glucose was still low, but returning to normal, John would say angry things to her, without any awareness of it, in front of the rescue team. When he was finally okay but not remembering the details, he could not understand why she was so angry with him. She felt unappreciated for being there for him. She was also embarrassed and angry that it seemed to be her fault that they had needed to call 911. Their relationship was deteriorating.

Each of them needed to do new things. John needed to mourn. He had not experienced any emotional reaction to his diabetes. He warded off these feelings by being compulsive in his adherence behavior. None of the health care professionals detected a problem because he actually looked like a perfect patient, absorbing every fact and coming out with normal long-term blood glucose readings (hemoglobin A_{1C}). He never mentioned to the doctors how frequent the rescue calls had become, because they were not really part of his anxiety. He had been out of it, due to the low blood glucose, and had not been the one to make the calls.

Joint marital sessions were a welcome relief for both of them. She let go of her guilt and anger when they both came in touch with the sadness and fear they felt about diabetes coming into their lives. Sara was concerned that John had stopped enjoying food and was upset about how nervous he was when he could not follow a rigid schedule. He had so many restrictions that he placed on both of them about timing, restaurants, and types of food, despite the medical team's encouragement to be flexible. She had tried to help by questioning him often. She began to realize that she gave him the message that she was only looking to hear answers that would make her comfortable. She just wanted him to change. John listened attentively to what she was saying.

He began his own work on how to be okay with depending on insulin. In retrospect, it was the diabetes and the angry feelings from the loss of control, not the need for insulin that was the most upsetting to him. He was touched that Sara was willing to conquer her fears and learn a very difficult thing on his behalf—giving glucagon injections. It was the renewed closeness in their relationship along with his wife's willingness to learn something new that eased him into trying on new perspectives about diabetes. He worked hard to see that he was actually depending on himself, to make good decisions about insulin. With this framework in mind, he focused on being flexible and letting the insulin do its work. Their relationship helped them both conquer their fears.

Barry, who has type 2 diabetes and uses insulin, was a member of a diabetes support group. One day, he brought in a note that his wife, Joan, wanted him to read to the group. "I am going crazy," it began, "and if you don't help me, I've a mind to kill Barry or myself. As you are hearing this, you have now become accomplices. He blames me and others for his low blood sugars. I can't decide if I should die from guilt or anger. Signed, Desperate in Chicago." She used a screen of humor, but it was clear that she was feeling despair. They were locked in a control struggle about Barry's increasing low blood sugars. As open as he appeared in the group, Barry had never discussed his feelings or reported the frequency of his low blood sugars. He had not mentioned the constant bickering with his wife, either.

Introducing Joan's needs, via the note she sent in, was immensely helpful not only for her but in assisting Barry to face feelings he would otherwise have neglected. That is one of the beauties of being in a relationship. We can see wonderful things and problem areas about ourselves when our partners point them out, things that we otherwise would have missed. It became a joke for the group that everyone had to bring in a note from home—spouses, parents, children—all were encouraged and accepted. It was a funny but also a valuable way for the partner's insights to be brought into the group.

This communication from Barry's wife fortunately opened up his long-suppressed anger about diabetes. He hated not feeling in control of what his body did. He said he felt himself purposefully pushing the limit, always trying to complete one more thing before he decided to treat his low blood glucose. As a result, he would always go very low, requiring help. He grew resentful that his wife had to help him and then nagged him about not taking care of himself. He became angry with her rather than focusing on the real target of his fury, the burdens and sense of dependency that diabetes—and especially low blood glucose—placed on him.

The situation is actually about Barry realistically fitting diabetes into his life. It is also about Joan choosing not to fix his denial, but rather to step back to see repeating behavior patterns and insist that Barry talk them through with her. By asking the group for help, and airing the feelings and conflicts, this was no longer a control struggle between them. With time, Barry worked out his struggle with diabetes. The primary problem was his attitude about the diabetes, not the diabetes itself.

GENDER ISSUES REVISITED

Being male or female can color the way you look at having diabetes and for your partner, the caregiver role. Sometimes men have difficulty adjusting to diabetes because it challenges their stereotypical sense of themselves—they need not to be vulnerable or require help. Women who have diabetes but have been socialized to nurture others and leave themselves for last are at risk of sacrificing good diabetes care.

Men and women, patient or partner, can learn to expand their gender roles to take care of their health and improve each other's quality of life. The male partner, particularly during periods when caregiving is needed, can stretch to focus on the emotional needs of his spouse and children. The female partner, if caregiving is necessary, can learn to feel competent about the traditional male tasks (finances, taking charge).

Truly, men and women can be valuable assets in helping each other grow. I learned a priceless lesson from my stepson Dean. I told him how upset I was with a male friend for how he had handled a professional situation for me. I was proud of my determination to call my friend and tell him exactly what had bothered me and how I felt he should have handled it. Surprised by what I was calling assertiveness, Dean offered his perspective and how he would have liked to hear my message of disappointment.

He suggested that I begin by simply saying that I wasn't pleased with the experience. If I did not get a response, then I might ask what his thoughts were on how to remedy the situation. Dean had explained that perhaps it was a guy thing, but that he liked feeling independent and self-reliant in his interactions, coming up with his own ideas on how to handle situations.

I discussed the differing needs of men and women with my other stepson Bruce. Taking a different tack from his brother, he laughingly said that men probably don't know what they need. Even if he denies saying that, he was profound in continuing on to say that men and women help each other grow by teaching each other things they are either unaware of or not good at. Assertiveness is not about anger, rather it's about expression and heart. That is the way men and women can tutor each other.

However, this only happens if you are not too intimidated to stay true to what you think and feel. Rejection of the help or intimacy you try to share does not mean that it is without worth or that it is not needed by the other person. The best favor you can give each other is to become self-confident and to tune in to your loved ones while you find ways to reach them, in their language and with respect for their boundaries.

The following are examples to give you a helpful framework: don't forget that these are stereotypes about communication goals and styles. We all find ourselves crossing back and forth and using different styles of communication with different people and situations. (For more information, see Deborah Tannen's *You Just Don't Understand*, and John Gray's *Men Are From Mars and Women Are From Venus.)*

Men and women are just different, not superior or inferior. And, they are different from these stereotypes. Despite the frustrations of trying to understand each other, we need to be careful not to become the correcting, nagging, controlling, withdrawing or disapproving "parent." Even if we find these new ways of relating difficult or something we don't believe in, we still need to try them on. Have patience. If you respond in ways that will actually make your partner happier, you will be hap-

Women	Men
Emotional support	Rational support
Listening, empathy, compassion	Solve problems, advise
Interdependence, relationships	Independence, self-reliance
Spend much time talking, asking questions, details	Efficiency (Keep talk and details to a minimum)
Tend to be sensitive	Not bothered easily
Conversation goal: closeness	Conversation goal: fix problems
Communication is staff of life	Feel okay without expressiveness, likes space
Talk and touch before and after sex	Sex, before and after (Forgive a stereotype joke)

pier too. Your efforts can start out as tools you use to be effective and then slowly become attitudes that are natural and genuine for you.

Combining an awareness of gender differences with the skills you have been working on all along can be a powerful combination. You can speak to each other clearly—mind-reading is out.

A woman with diabetes might be talking to her partner about how hard it is for her to refuse a mid-morning snack at work. In response to his natural response, "Then don't eat," (rational, advice-giving) she will whine that he never listens and doesn't care about her. (sensitive) The consequences of receiving advice too quickly is feeling dependent, embarrassed, or incompetent. If he thinks about different gender needs, he will speak to her while looking her in the eye and touching her hand. "I can hear why it feels so hard for you not to eat." (listening and empathy) Or, "Tell me some more—not too much more (kidding)—about why it is so difficult for you." (emotional support and questioning) She will more likely feel loved and cared about, and feel generous in return. Further, she will feel more capable and more likely come up with an independent solution. That's how he can be a partner in solving her problem with her.

In response to a partner who is giving advice and trying to cheer you up, (rational, solving problems) you could become angry and annoyed and critical. With gender awareness under your belt, you can say instead, "I just want to express my feelings. (communication for closeness) Please don't talk me out of them, not yet, anyway. I need you, but for now, I need you just to listen. Thanks, in advance, for trying something new."

Or, in response to a partner who shouted at you that you are always pushing him to talk, you might have been defensive and yelled back a put-down. Now, armed with awareness, and respect for his way of seeing things, you might say, "Yes, I can see why it seems to you that I am nagging you." **(nondefensive** and **empathy)** WAIT FOR AN ANSWER. If there is not a response, you can continue. "Maybe first I should ask if you are ready to talk." WAIT AGAIN. "If you aren't ready to talk now, I'd like to choose a time with you when you will." **(assertive**

questioning) "I have a sneaking suspicion you might like talking to me if I could keep it shorter and ask fewer questions." (independence, efficiency)

Yes, it is artificial. But that is only until it becomes a good habit for you to speak in a manner that slices out defensiveness and hostility. Because all people really have different needs, you can modify your conversations to fit the other's style. This is not done to be subservient, but rather to show self-respect, respect for the other, and to be effective. People are more willing to stretch the ways they relate if they see that you are trying, too. Men, if it doesn't work to offer advice, don't offer advice. Women, if it turns him off to have you asking how he feels, give it up and find a different route.

Siblings without Diabetes

Some truths stand the test of time. For your parents to make sure there is enough energy left over for all the children in the family after taking care of diabetes is not easy. And no matter what age you and your siblings are, your relationship is complex, often filled with rivalry, jealousy, power struggles, or anger. Another truth that you may not realize, or admit to at times, is that the positives about your brothers and sisters far outweigh the negatives. The sibling relationship offers you a unique opportunity for the development of intimacy and honesty that children don't have with their parents or even their friends.

Tommy remembers he was about 8 years old when his older brother Ted, 10, was diagnosed with diabetes. It is not easy for Tommy to look back at that period. There were so many difficult feelings, most of which, unfortunately, he felt ashamed of having. Tommy never shared what he was thinking and feeling with anyone at the time. There was really no one to talk to; everyone was absorbed in Ted. He had always idolized and loved his older brother, but those feelings were overshadowed by losing his special place, the youngest who was adored by everyone.

Tommy began to feel desperate for attention, yet he knew he should not get in the way or cause more problems because his parents had enough worry, figuring out all the details of his brother's diabetes. Sometimes he was so lonely and angry, he felt like running away. He wouldn't actually do anything like that because he couldn't upset them or let them down any more than they already were. Maybe if he was really good, really achieved a lot, his parents might give him some special consideration, too. He tried harder and harder but doing well was never enough to change the focus toward him. And worse still was the fact that his doing well made him feel guilty that he was surpassing his brother who was always missing school and falling behind.

He gave up on trying to get attention for himself, shifting his role to one of accommodating everyone in the family and remaining on the periphery. Sometimes it would get to him that he was like an outsider in the home where he had once enjoyed sharing center stage. Sometimes he would feel angry with his brother and his parents, but that would quickly turn to shame when his mother would say to him how lucky she was to have such an easy kid. Sometimes he felt that underneath he was an awful person, trying to take time away from his brother who had difficulties enough with the diabetes.

No one noticed the difficulty Tommy was having until ninth grade, when an especially observant teacher noticed that while he did well in school, he seemed slightly depressed. They got to talking, and the teacher was able to empathize with him because he, too, had grown up with a sibling who had a chronic illness. The teacher told him he had handled it differently, as a kid. He was always getting into trouble, hoping to get noticed. The two bonded, and eventually Tommy gave the teacher permission to talk with his parents and try to get him some help with revising his role in the family.

The family went to counseling together, which relieved all of them. Everyone in the family was unhappy about how their lives were going. Diabetes had taken over more than it needed to. Ted liked the attention in some ways, but the constant focus on him also felt intrusive and demeaning. As a result, he was impatient and short-tempered most of the time. He missed talking and playing with Tommy and thought Tommy's indifference to him was rejection. Their mother was burned out and irritable in her interactions with Ted, always saying he wasn't doing something well enough, and guilty about not giving enough time to her husband and Tommy. Their father was upset that the adults had no time together and was getting home later and later, causing tension because he was not helping with the kids or the household. It was a good thing that Tommy's issues were picked up. Intervention helped the entire family get back to living life in more satisfying ways without shortchanging Ted's health status.

1. Does any part of Tommy's story sound familiar?
2. Do you find any of these things happening to you or your family members?
3. How has diabetes changed your life?
4. Has your family become closer?
5. Are there more arguments?
6. Do you like the way your family lives together or do you wish some things were different?

DEAR BROTHERS AND SISTERS

Hopefully, you can talk to your family about what you are feeling. Be prepared, though, that they may be upset at first, and give them time to think, and if necessary, to cool off. You'll be glad to get it off your chest and the important thing is to get started. It can take a while to change your routines together. You can always ask your doctor for some additional help.

You are important to your family, but you need more than just to know that in your heart. You need people to act that way with you. It is not selfish for you to want the same attention that your sister or brother has; it is normal. Sometimes you do have to take a back seat, but not all the time. Diabetes isn't all emergencies and crises.

You can do the things you want to do and still be a good friend to your sister or brother. If you want to eat junk food or all the Halloween candy in one sitting, but your sibling isn't, you can probably work out a compromise that takes care of you and shows kindness and understanding to him or her. Ask to be part of the decisions around food, so you can feel included and proud of yourself when you're eating healthfully, too (or pleased that you are considerate and making good choices, not just being obedient). A satisfying sibling relationship is important for your own positive self-image. You can try on all sorts of behaviors and learn valuable lessons from the positive and negative feedback that you get from each other. These experiences help you grow up well rounded and healthy.

There are at least two additional things for you to think about. First, how can you get enough nurturing attention to avoid feeling neglected, getting into trouble, or becoming a depressed martyr? Second, what positive role can you play in your sister or brother's life with diabetes? Your role is special. Your parents worry, others may be afraid of the diabetes, but you can treat your brother or sister as normal. What a welcome relief!

SIBLING RIVALRY

Sometimes it feels like there is not enough love to go around. Don't be afraid of jealousy, resentment, or anger that may overcome you at times. These feelings are all a part of sibling rivalry. Hopefully, your parents remind you that you are lovable even when you have difficult feelings. Sibling rivalry has been around a long time; check out the Bible. This is a natural competition for your parents' attention and for each other's approval. In fact, rivalry has something good to offer you—self-control, experience in competition, assertiveness, and a sense of knowing your limits. This comes with love, loyalty, and mutual protection for each other. See the rich potential in your sibling relationship?

Rivalry gone astray, however, does some damage. At the 1997 meeting of the American Psychological Association, researchers warned that parents should not allow siblings to heap emotional and verbal abuse—ridicule, slurs, indignities, shaming—on each other. Verbal abuse had lasting negative effects on children. The other side of the coin is that not only can you hurt each other, but you can truly help each other, too. You can be a positive influence on your sibling and the course of the diabetes, and your good works can boost your own self-esteem and people skills.

GOOD NEWS

You may actually be getting enough attention. Perhaps you just haven't realized it. The trade-off for you, if you are getting less attention at times, is that you have opportunities to grow in self-confidence, patience, loyalty, tolerance, empathy, resilience, independence, and thoughtfulness. You need to feel you are part of the hard work and are appreciated for your personal sacrifice. Maybe if you start recognizing all the things that other people do and compliment them, they'll see what you do and thank you, too.

TOUGH STUFF

You probably are experiencing some difficult situations that families without diabetes are not exposed to with such intensity or at such an early age. You may feel anger at the increased responsibility, particularly when you are an older child taking care of a younger sibling. You may feel vulnerable, fearing for your own health—will you get diabetes, too? (There is testing that may help determine your degree of risk for diabetes.) You may feel lonely that no one understands your new position, embarrassed that others may tease you or your sibling, resentment over more lenient discipline for your sibling, guilt (especially from kids under age 7 who have "magical thinking," that is that you can cause bad things just by thinking them). You may feel a sense of survivor guilt or guilt that you don't have diabetes, too.

Jim, age 35, has had type 1 diabetes for 27 years and recalls that he was always taunted before dinner by his two older brothers, mocking him for his moodiness. "Let's take bets," they'd say, "on what mood Jim comes to dinner in. Will he be grouchy or nasty? Those are our choices." Then they would laugh together, sharing their private joke. It was one more way that Jim felt different and isolated with his diabetes. His mother was always anxiously telling him that he must tell everyone, not because he had nothing to hide or be ashamed of, but in case something bad happened and people would have to watch out for him. This added to his defensive, inferior, helpless feeling. Jim always hid his diabetes from friends because he was not going to risk being vulnerable or judged by friends as he was by his family.

One day, in a support group, watching the siblings of some of the younger children, it hit him. His brothers had been jealous of all the extra attention and easier double standard he received from their mother. They probably had no other outlet for venting their jealousy and resentment of him. If only he had understood then that their rejection and putdowns were not about the diabetes but the favoritism, he might have been able to stop concealing and being embarrassed about having diabetes. That was a lot to think and talk about.

Your feelings and your interactions with each other and your parents will range over a wide spectrum, depending on personalities, whether you are male or female, older or younger, and even the size of your family.

You have completed your first step of getting in touch with your feelings. The second step is to accept your feelings (not be ashamed of them) and to try to understand them. (For more information, see chapter 3 on coping.)

WHAT WOULD YOU FEEL?

You see your younger brother with diabetes eating two candy bars in a row, looking furtively around, making sure no one sees him. You feel:

- sympathetic to how difficult some things are for him
- disinterested, it is his life
- excited that you will be able to tell on him (he has been getting too much attention lately, anyway)
- anxious that you should say something
- guilty if you don't say something
- dread at the upcoming conversation (he gets so angry lately)
- tired of being the older brother with two working parents, having to take over your brother's supervision, which is more than you think is fair

You say:

To your brother: It must be awfully hard to always have to think about what you are eating when it seems like no one else is. **(assertive empathy)** I want to help you when it is particularly tough to do it by yourself. How can I do that without being a pain in the neck? **(assertive request)**

To your parents: Mayday. Mayday. I need some help here. Could I get a day off from playing Poppa Bear so I can feel young and foolish? Would that knock me off the list of your favorite children?

This is mature of you. You use humor to express your concern that you might lose their love. You don't improve your image by showing your brother's mistakes. You need the attention that is rightfully yours and the normal amount of freedom necessary.

Of course no one really talks like that. I know, I am trying to set a standard here that may not be natural but is worth trying. It definitely beats the alternative of just hitting back.

PRACTICE MAKES PERFECT

Parent to sibling: Can't you be nicer to Johnny? You know he is not feeling well. Please do the dishes for him, he is going to go lie down.

Response: I don't want to be rude, Mom, but I will feel much nicer to Johnny if I am not always having to pick up his slack. (assertive) We both know he will feel better soon; thank goodness it is just a low blood sugar. Maybe he can do the dishes in a while, and I will sit and talk to him while he does them to make sure he is okay. (assertive empathy and request)

ADULT SIBLINGS

The emotions are probably not quite as intense when your sibling gets diagnosed with type 2 diabetes as an adult, but many of the same feelings can arise. Attention from the parent for adult children can still elicit resentment if it is meted out unevenly. If there are no parents alive among adult children, sibling issues still have a pulse.

Howard was age 51 and overweight with type 2 diabetes. Since the death of their mother, one of his younger sisters, Jennifer, age 49, had taken over the mothering role and aggressively mounted campaigns for him to lose weight and exercise. His sister had even gone so far as to offer to pay for a personal trainer for him, to get him started. Howard was furious. There were complex reasons for his anger.

Howard resented Jennifer giving advice, mothering him, or offering help. It was not about the money—Howard had enough to pay for his own personal trainer. It was not about being judged or feeling inferior. His sister had battled weight her entire life and was certainly at risk for getting diabetes, too. But he had been the caretaker brother growing up, so he felt wounded and defensive at the idea that he needed any help. He also had a diagnosed depression that sabotaged his taking any positive action on changing his life by himself. Now, with his sister's interference, the bad feelings seemed to expand.

Howard was lost in negatives. He saw his sister's offer as demeaning, intrusive, and controlling. He thought she was really self-centered, thinking she wanted him to do well just to please her. This put a burden of expectations and obligations on him. It reminded him of how his mother had so often made the children feel their successes were about pleasing her, rather than themselves. His opposition and pessimistic focus was too narrow. He saw an exercise regimen as giving up something—a superior role or his sense of independence—to his younger sister, rather than what it needed to be—part of his own goal for good self-care. He could actually see himself turning his back on his own health so he wouldn't give in to what someone else wanted for him. Ironically, this meant that his sister was controlling his behavior—just negatively.

Sibling relationships are complex. Jennifer loved her brother. They were very close, and her feelings were intensified by his having been a parent figure for her. It is healthy for siblings occasionally to "mother" each other, but it should be flexible, not constant. In this case, Jennifer had great anxiety that she would lose Howard if he didn't take care of his diabetes. She was just trying to help him, not boss him. She knew he was in control of what he chose to do and diabetes was his responsibility. Her manner may have had some roots in her position as youngest in the family, needing to give advice to be validated as a worthwhile person.

Basically, however, her motivation for wanting her brother to be well might be tagged healthy selfishness. She could say to him, "Of course, I would be happier if you exercised. You are more fun when you are feeling good." This would not remind him of what he should do but of what gave him pleasure before diabetes came along—feeling well through exercising and eating healthfully. Her tone of voice must be relaxed as in casual conversation. She could face his resentment of her by saying, "I need some conversation on this matter. You might bite my head off and reject what I am saying, but I hope that on some level it will register on you. I can't make you change, but I would like you to know that I care about you. I wish good things for you and sometimes feel agitated about it all." Regardless of her skillful attempts to interact, Howard refused to accept it as a generous and loving message. He was irritated by Jennifer's request that he see the impact his health status had on her. It didn't matter what she wished for him. He was not yet ready to acknowledge his own self-centeredness.

As in the chapters on families and couples, siblings also have conflict over their styles and levels of intimacy. They have to find a balance between too much detachment, healthy detachment (caring and respect for the other), and intrusion (trying to take control). Each family achieves this balance in their individual ways.

Depression occurs more often in people with diabetes and it is often the family members who are the first to identify it and encourage treatment. Depression is not caused by character flaws or weakness. The roots are often biological and need professional treatment. You can cause conflict in your family when you point out the symptoms and suggest treatment. You have to have emotional stamina to bear the denial and anger you may receive in return. Howard and I worked together to understand why he resisted getting help. He wanted changes to come totally from himself and to be in control of it all. Many adults do not like needing help. How long would he let his false pride and wanting to be independent at any price endanger his health? What did he have to win in that situation?

Howard needed to take the first step and admit that he alone could not find the power to make a change, in a 12-step-type program, *without feeling diminished by it*. His fears and stubbornness were controlling him. Admitting powerlessness can actually open a door to new approaches. An Alcoholics Anonymous slogan—Action Precedes Understanding—suggests people need to do some things first, without understanding all the details. This is difficult for those who live by their intellects, because it feels like they're giving up control. What actually happens is that trying something new helps to overcome the fears and breaks the deadlock.

The medical team and therapists sometimes use a concept of "lending the ego." In effect, you give a hand to the individual, saying, "Trust me for now. Try on my sense of caring about your reality. You are stuck in a spot where you cannot find your strength or discipline. Diabetes has undercut your adult sense of independence. Now, you have to depend on insulin and doctors. Even though you don't want to take care of yourself, have faith in my judgment, and do these things. Stick with me. Let me be the decision maker until you find the will to continue on your own." Siblings can be involved in lending the ego too.

How siblings get involved is important. Nagging, judging, and criticism are out. Be respectful.

JEALOUSY CAN GO BOTH WAYS

Feelings of jealousy or being left out do not spring only from the sibling without diabetes. Children with diabetes can be envious of your wellness, your spontaneity, and your freedom to eat whatever you want, without other people watching what you do. They, too, feel anger and resentment that you seem to have more privileges, no one monitors or restricts you, and you don't have to cope with feeling different. They can get lost in their feelings, and not think about what it is like for you. Some adults with type 2 have told us that as they watch their overweight brothers or sisters freely eating whatever they want, they feel both jealousy over this liberty to eat and protective concern that the siblings are placing themselves at risk of getting diabetes. They feel reluctant to share warnings, assuming they'll be accused of just being jealous. So they stay silent and don't help prevent the type 2 diabetes that might occur in their relatives.

Reneé, a 12-year-old girl with diabetes, was in the hospital for diabetic ketoacidosis. Her parents had just been through a bitter divorce. All the children were unhappy about it. Reneé's diabetes was affected by the emotional stress, the beginning of adolescence, her own sabotaging of the diabetes, and less supervision by her parents. It was the father's weekend to be with the kids. The other siblings were very young and could not stay long in the hospital, so the father took them out to lunch. Reneé was furious at her father for letting them have a good time while she was suffering in the hospital. Feeling guilty, anyway, about the hospitalization, the father, regrettably, snapped at her, saying she was selfish to think that way and that her diabetes had taken much time from all of them.

Reneé didn't need to be ashamed of her feelings. Neither did her sisters and brothers need to stay home without special attention. It was a difficult situation for all of them. In frustration, guilt, and exhaustion, the father missed an opportunity to accept her feelings and to make a point to himself and Reneé about how they both could help her achieve better self-care.

ATTITUDES TOWARD GETTING ATTENTION

Some children look for appreciation by not taking up time, which may help them be self-sufficient in self-care but doesn't get adequate acknowledgment for their needs. Others may try to compensate for an imbalance of attention by getting attention for disruptive behavior or by being perfect—a burden for a young person either way. Diabetes may split the parents or get parents thinking that the nondiabetic child is the one to push.

One 30-year-old sibling, Sandra, felt angry that she was encouraged to do more things because her sister Anne had brittle diabetes and was not allowed to do many things. Sandra felt like she was living for two. She found it difficult to enjoy things because they seemed to be for others, not for herself. Even her decision to have children was for her parents and sister. When her marriage was not working, she was afraid to make changes, feeling she would be letting everyone down.

Depression brought Sandra and eventually the entire family came into counseling. In facing her own feelings, Sandra tapped Anne's anger. Anne had felt discounted and overlooked, except when she was actually sick, so she used the pattern of getting attention through illness. She said she frequently omitted her insulin so she could be hospitalized when she was a child. As an adult, Anne found it difficult to change her sickly image and find satisfaction from normal things.

The birth of a younger sibling, in any family, is grounds for jealousy over your special spot being taken. If your younger sibling gets diabetes, it takes away even more time from you. If you are older without diabetes, you might be protective and act like another parent. Your sex also may impact your status in the family; sometimes sons are favored over daughters, despite who has diabetes.

Even as you grow older and try to make the relationships more equal, there still exists an age hierarchy. The eldest may need to retain that role. Often the younger siblings are not aware of their own power or that their older siblings need to have the younger ones approve of them. In cases where the oldest has diabetes as an adult, younger siblings sometimes feel hesitant to give advice or encouragement and feel surprised that they may actually have any influence on them. The conflicts between siblings are often not expressed directly but instead acted out by others close to them.

Susan, 60 years old, has an older sister Lauren, 65 with type 2 diabetes, who denies the significance of her diabetes and does not take care of herself or make efforts to get help. As the younger sister, Susan has been unable to feel that she has the right to talk to her older sister about what may happen to her. Even though she is involved successfully in her own family, she needs for her big sister to stay strong and healthy—a feeling left over from childhood. She would like to share her compassion, "I think all the time about how hard this must be for you," and her concerns, "I am so concerned, knowing that your mismanagement may lead to an early death or complications."

Because she feels unable to challenge her sister, Susan remains upset with her and wavers between feeling loving and feeling cold and distant. She feels powerless. Susan was also bothered by intense negative feelings toward her brother-in-law, though she never really understood why until she started to talk about it in therapy. He, by marriage to her older sister, was also an authority figure for Susan. This made her doubly upset with him because he didn't move her sister toward better health practices. She began to understand that she projected her own failure to influence her sister onto her brother-in-law, as well.

Susan sees that she and the brother-in-law are frustrated at being unable to stop her sister, and they seem to move from being silent or angry "enablers" to giving up their efforts at trying to control her. Sarcasm and criticism seldom get creative change started. Realistically, the only thing that Susan can control in this situation is how she chooses to feel about her sister's choices or the conversations they have.

Neither sister can change the other. They can share their feelings and their love and try to empathize with each other. Susan can say, "I will always be there for you. Maybe you will be open to talk about it again. I'm sad for you if you can't make the changes you want. I certainly empathize with how hard this must be for you. It is painful to see you hurting yourself. When I know you are getting professional help, I feel glad for you. When you go through your periods of avoiding professional help, I want to avoid you, too." Susan can also forge an alliance with her brother-in-law for mutual support and to offer effective, honest, and concrete support that Lauren certainly needs to help her get started.

Family members who stop talking directly, out of loving concern, about neglect of care are similar to physicians who don't discuss that their patients need to stop smoking during each visit. (Many patients tell me their physicians don't care that much about it because they only mentioned it on the first visit.) Their impact on Lauren will be in helping to empower her through conversation and support rather than "fixing" her. Their personal sense of power can only be found in their own lives.

PREVENTION

If you are a sibling of someone with type 2 diabetes, the greatest gift to yourself (and to your sibling) is to live your life in a healthy manner and be a wonderful role model.

Other Significant Others: Grandparents, Teachers, Friends, and Baby-sitters

Grandparents, aunts, uncles, friends, teachers, baby-sitters, lend me your ears. You know you have a significant place in the life of someone with diabetes. All that has been said in other chapters applies to relationships in general and so to you. Understanding diabetes is difficult. Perhaps you would like to know more. Some of you would like to know less. Believe me, you are in good company. Your loved ones wish they didn't have to know that much, either. With effort and time, your uncomfortable feelings will subside, and you will have the generosity of spirit to help them face difficult situations and feelings.

WHAT CAN YOU DO?

The rewards of gathering knowledge and being helpful to the family may not be obvious to you or them, at first. It is a wonderful gesture of support to arm yourself with concrete information for the people you care about. When you know about diabetes or express interest in learning more, you gain access to conversations that you could not otherwise have with the person who has diabetes. Through all my years of working with people, I have seen how touched they are when someone is interested and knowledgeable about diabetes.

If you choose to be involved, then bring all the skills you would to any relationship and a bit more. People with diabetes spend a lot of time being poked and prodded with needles and questions. They have been at the receiving end of authority in most of their interactions and have an exquisite sensitivity to being told what to do.

Part of supporting another person is being honest about your observations at times. When things are not going well, this information may not be well received but is nonetheless valuable. Sharing some loving, nonjudgmental dialogue can be compared to not letting a friend drive home drunk.

THINGS YOU CAN DO

1. Be interested and knowledgeable.
2. Give feedback, not criticism. Point out the positives, not the negatives.
4. Ask questions. They are the experts.
5. Be empathetic and compassionate.
6. Pick good timing for discussions.
7. Work on your own issues (be a good role model).
8. Support and be a part of the reward system.
9. Don't give up. See nonadherence as temporary and encourage restarting.

GRANDPARENT POWER

Being a grandparent is a special opportunity. The joys of this very unique relationship emphasize mutual love and acceptance. This is a relationship that is mostly about enjoying each other. Because this is the second time around for grandparents, in terms of understanding a child's needs, they are usually more tolerant, patient, and ready to share pragmatic wisdom.

In a support group that I lead, there is a set of grandparents who touch my heart. Their grandson, an 18-year-old with diabetes, lives 1000 miles away. They do not have to take care of him during a visit because the grandson is self-sufficient. That is not the reason they come to the meetings. It is their way of saying, if someone we love so much has something difficult to handle, we want to understand it, find out about the latest research, and be able to communicate with him about the details. It also salves the grandparents' heartache to get support from others. Their hearts are still too heavy with sadness for their family to realize the admiration they receive from the group. Some of the parents of children with diabetes lament that their own parents are not a part of their children's lives in such an active, loving way. Many are inspired to reach out again to try to get them more involved.

Sometimes, for varying reasons, grandparents don't offer to learn and be closely involved in caring for or understanding their grandchildren's health. My advice to parents is that if their parents don't initiate active participation, then they must ask for it and show the grandparents how to become comfortable with the child's diabetes. What may feel like rejection is, in most cases, honest cowardice more than selfishness, and sometimes a gentle nudge is all that's needed. Sometimes, however, this is not enough. It's easy to understand the resistance. If you didn't have to do it, how many of you would?

If you love the child or take part in caring for him, then you do have to. You don't want to give a message of "I love you, except for your diabetes."

AUNTS, UNCLES, AND ALL OTHER RELATIVES, TOO

It is important for aunts, uncles, and cousins to get involved. Learn about nutrition, exercise, the part stress plays, insulin, and low blood glucose. Information gives you power over fear and brings the family closer together. It is lonely for people with diabetes to have only a few people who understand the issues and tactics that pepper their daily lives.

At the very least, the child's relationship with relatives usually includes sleepovers or week-long vacations, and this should not change because of diabetes.

DOING THE DIFFICULT TASKS

I see 70-year-old adults with diabetes learn to give themselves injections, despite trepidation, so I know that physically grandparents can learn. The emotional part is more difficult. You don't want to see a child that you love have to go through something so troublesome. It is also frightening that while in your care, your grandchild may have high blood glucose or low blood glucose—both natural events that happen at home and school, too.

What is the worst that can happen? Nothing that a little food, or a little insulin, or at the very worse, a call to 911 can't fix, and quickly at that. Through the years, plenty of parents have called their medical teams to say they accidentally overdosed their child with too much insulin. Health care providers are a hotline helping families through the extra testing and eating that needs to be done. I am not minimizing the importance of what you have to know and do or the risks, but I certainly will not maximize fears, particularly if they get in the way of you being close and loving.

Let's go over a few situations that raise difficult issues for everyone. If you try to imagine yourself on each side of the interaction, you can be more compassionate for the other person, something that helps soften fear or anger. (See chapter 3 for coping skills.)

> **Grandparent:** It is too hard for me to give my grandson the insulin shot. I will drop him off before dinner.
>
> **Parent:** I know what you mean. I felt exactly the same way when Johnny was diagnosed. **(normalizing** and **empathy)** I think you can get used to it. It would mean a lot to Johnny and me if you give it a try, and then he can stay overnight the way he used to. Would you come with me on Wednesday to see the nurse, who can go over the details with you? **(assertive request)**

I know you had to bite your tongue to get to this place if you interpreted your parents' reaction as selfishness, rejection, or lack of interest. You have made a good start. You are helping them help you. You are being honest about what you want to happen and not focusing only on feeling injured or angry.

Keeping this conversation from going straight downhill was not easy. A fight with your own mother, with all the pressure already on you, is not something you need. Many people tend to criticize when they are concerned. That is what the grandparent did in this example. Notice

Grandparent: I think you are too loose with Johnny. You let him eat whatever he wants.

Parent: I think you mean to be helpful. **(positive reframing)** Your comment is hurtful to me and not really accurate. It would support Johnny and me if you would learn some of the new and flexible ideas they are teaching us about choosing foods. I could use some help with figuring out how to set limits without feeling guilty. **(assertive request)** I know diabetes is a big worry for you, too. **(empathy)**

how the adult child's speaking honestly to the issue enabled her/him to find some empathy by the end of the conversation for the grandparent. Each person is hurting here, and they could all use mutual support. If the situation were reversed and the parent was telling the grandparent that she was not going to let her son stay overnight anymore because he always came home with his blood glucose out of whack, they would need the same compassion for each other's frustration with a difficult task.

The use of positive reframing gives you time not to succumb to the child's suggestion and keeps you from

Grandchild: I promise to go to bed on time if you just let me eat three more cookies.

Grandparent: Clever kid. Now that is a creative way to get a cookie. **(positive reframing)** Are you still hungry? Can you figure out a plan for tonight or tomorrow that lets you enjoy some cookies *and* good blood sugars? **(assertive request)** Your mother used to try to bargain with me over food, too, when she was a kid. **(normalizing)**

being angry at a normal request from your grandchild. Wanting more cookies is a birthright, not necessarily having anything to do with diabetes. Your grandchild does not have to be ashamed of being a normal kid, trying to get away with what he can. Being able to say a simple no without judgment is the skill here.

FRIENDS

In other chapters, we discuss the importance of friends in taking care of diabetes. We never outgrow our need for friends. Lois Wyse has an inscription in her book *Women Make the Best Friends* that says, "For the friends life has given me, and for the life friends have given me." That sums up nicely the support, solace, motivation, and feedback that friends give to us, helping us enjoy our good times, assisting us in getting through our crises, and taking risks to help us grow. A researcher from Purdue University, Brant Burleson, suggests that the best way to help a friend with a crisis is to ask him/her to talk about the problem and his/her feelings in detail. This is more helpful than you stepping in with similar stories, giving advice, trying to distract them, or even trying to find the positive in the situation.

I met Sandy Bernstein when we were 22 years old. Within 20 minutes of our initial introduction, we were deep in the excited chatter that the chemistry of friendship can bring. Twenty-eight years later, we are still laughing and talking, no matter where we are. When it came time for me to confront my fears about writing this book, I asked her to be the first person to read it. "A friend is someone who knows all about you and likes you, anyway." She has read every word, chapter by chapter, and has been supporter and generous critic. If I had diabetes, I could sit down with her and go over my blood glucose records, being honest about the trouble spots I did not have courage or patience to correct.

So if one of your friends has diabetes, that person exposes you to healthy habits and some special personal qualities. People in the process of mastering their diabetes have had to develop tolerance for disappointment, problem-solving skills, a certain depth and sensitivity, and an appreciation for good times and good people. People faced with the vulnerability of contemplating their health and looking at their mortality are often very good at living in the present. Those are nice traits to find in friends.

Remember that people with diabetes come by their defenses honestly. A child with diabetes needs to figure out a way to deal with all the comments about diabetes that can hurt his or her feelings from "Yuk!" (an honest children's response), to "Oh, no, how awful for such a young person." There are many people who comment on the diabetes, often uninvited and with ignorance, even if well-meaning. Most people with diabetes are forced to listen to terrible stories about someone's grandmother's diabetes. The child must find an exterior demeanor that works and protects his self-esteem. The best response, of course, is nondefensive, just the calm persistence of a confident, centered individual, who does not let the opinions of other people upset or sway him or her.

Some people with diabetes have an outer layer of anger that they use for protection. They and their friends have to be alert to this defense mechanism, so they do not alienate each other or lose out on the benefits of friendships. My niece, Jennifer, taught me something the other day during one of our infrequent arguments. We were lovingly snapping at one another, and I was doing my usual (not necessarily good) talk-to-me-now routine. She bowled me over with her thoughtful response. "I want to cool off before I speak to you about this. I do not want my anger to become one of our problems." By her choice, she avoided an unpleasant experience for both of us.

People with type 2 diabetes probably have lifelong habits about food or exercise that are difficult to change. This has caused them inner turmoil, conflict, self-judgment, and feelings of failure. It is understandable that while you may feel you have the right or responsibility to discuss health issues, you must appreciate the exquisite sensitivity that has surrounded your friend with diabetes and be forgiving if s/he responds with great anger. Motivation is not something anyone is born with, and it waxes and wanes for all of us.

Make your intentions clear and pay attention to time and place in your interactions, and things will go more smoothly. My own friends have left the table during some of my attempts at conversations about their health. You learn pretty quickly what doesn't work. The trick is not to be scared off permanently.

FORGIVING FRIENDS

One of the really important qualities in friendships is the ability to forgive ourselves and each other. Whether we are children or adults, it is so easy to feel hurt by our friends for not being attentive enough or acting too much like mother hens. On the giving end, friends can be disappointed they do not get enough acknowledgment for the efforts they make. When we are hurt by friends who let us down, accidentally or intentionally, we have a choice. We can get lost in self-pity and remain isolated, resentful, or harbor thoughts of revenge. Keeping bitterness in our hearts negatively affects our health and our habits. The other choice—to forgive—shows true inner strength and frees us to continue to share friendship. It also has a profound effect on our health. Be humble. If you could understand things from your friend's point of view, you would probably not be hurt or mad. If your friend can't apologize, you can forgive in your heart to rid yourself of debilitating anger.

Sometimes when friends continually tell you how badly they are doing and how they are not putting effort into changing things or their attitudes, you need a different approach for your sake and theirs. You can ask, "What should I do with this information that you don't take care of yourself?" or "Are you interested in making it different for yourself?" or "I care about you. Here comes an observation, not a criticism. It is hard to listen, year after year, when you don't do anything about your health. I am not saying it is easy; I, too, have plenty of things that need working on. I just need to have different conversations with you about your health that are not about you being helpless and putting off changes."

Back off if a patient or friend says clearly, "I know what I am doing. I know what can happen to me. I know how badly I feel everyday physically from the high blood sugars. I have no guilt and no worry. I am making a clear choice." If they have not expressed this sentiment, and they are not taking care of themselves, they may actually be—no offense intended—temporarily insane and very much in need of friends.

HOW YOU DO IT

The how of involvement is easier to describe. Have empathy, respect the other person, and pace your information. Give up nagging or repetition, reinforce any positive changes in ideas or behaviors, and talk about future success (not past failure).

TEACHERS AND SCHOOL PERSONNEL

You are the significant group who gives the first objective feedback to a child or adolescent with or without diabetes. You are powerful shapers of children's feelings about themselves by your response and the atmosphere you build for the attitudes of the students toward each other. You have probably enjoyed and been apprehensive with this profound responsibility. I suggest the same thing to you as I do their parents—create a balance where you are appropriately protective and don't lower your expectations.

The stories kids have told me have made me understand the tremendous pressures on teachers and the family when a young person has diabetes. You have your own fears and questions about diabetes, and it will serve you best to have them addressed by the families or their health care professionals. You need to recognize *their* particular priorities in handling diabetes. The American Diabetes Association has information on what school personnel need to know. If you are interested, you are a joy, not a bother. Thank you for the efforts that you have made and will continue to make on behalf of these children.

Kids have told me wonderful stories about teachers who take the extra step of being interested and kind. They have also told me about other teachers who stare at them, watch everything they eat, and call their names out in class in front of other students to see if they are all right, while they die quietly of embarrassment. I certainly understand where those teachers are coming from. They are sincere, interested, adjusting, overprotective, and letting fear get in the way of their better judgment about handling children's feelings.

Then there are loving, overinvolved teachers whose well-meaning generosity turns into leniency and letting students do less than they could. They don't chide the student about missing class, but look empathetic, cocking their heads off to the side. They are the ones who let the student turn papers in late, knowing s/he has a lot to do. While that may be appropriate sometimes, it definitely hurts more than it helps if it becomes a pattern. Chronic special treatment can lead to fewer successes and keep a child from realizing how talented or skilled s/he actually is.

Even when you are committed to helping, sometimes you will feel a defensive reaction from parents and children. Identify yourself as an ally, a team member, when you need to share an observation that will help the child perform to full capacity. You may not have all the information you need about certain situations. Asking questions and listening well along with your observations can be so helpful.

Some school personnel are angry at the additional responsibility a child with diabetes brings to their jobs. This is usually the case at the beginning of the year before there is a relationship with the child and his family. Diabetes takes energy from teachers. They may not want to learn about the diabetes because of fear or just being overwhelmed by their regular duties. It is easy for children and families to feel angry and hurt by school personnel who seem insensitive. Time, patience, education, and communication are necessary before school personnel will become comfortable and knowledgeable about diabetes.

DIABETES TOOLS

Insulin and syringes are tools for health. The medical team encourages independence and safety for the child by requesting they carry around their own blood glucose meter, syringes, snacks, or glucose tablets. Section 504 of the Rehabilitation Act provides that children with diabetes can have individualized plans to help them take care of their health and not interfere with school. My interpretation of that means we give children permission to carry with them whatever is necessary for their health. We do not want to chip away at the self-esteem and anxiety levels of children by isolating and stigmatizing them or by not letting them take care of their own medical needs. It takes time to focus on the idea that syringes and the back of the room for privacy are special needs for wellness, not sickness. These are not sick kids who need to go to the clinic. These are healthy kids who have to do special things to be well.

OBSERVING THE PATTERNS

What you see the child do in the classroom may help his parents make diabetes care decisions. This might include observing the child leaving the room frequently to use the bathroom. Frequent need to urinate may mean high blood glucose, stemming from a number of causes. In diabetes, nothing is as simple as it seems. This information is helpful to parents who have to make a choice from a broad range such as needing more insulin in the mornings or helping a child to make better choices about food during lunch, or simply recognizing a cold or flu coming on that is raising blood glucose. All of this must be done without judgment. If you catch yourself feeling that the child is manipulating you, it is time to step back for compassion and setting some limits.

Another pattern that is helpful to note (not judge) is a child's appearing to have low blood glucose before every school test. These children are not only dealing with the anxiety of being prepared for the test but they may also worry about having high or low blood glucose during the test. It is possible that a child may think they are low and actually be high (or vice versa). Anxiety may legitimately feel like low blood glucose for many children and if it is mistakenly recognized as such, presents a different problem. Children with diabetes are probably more tuned-in to their bodies than most children and, while guidelines have been set, the kids must be a part of deciding what works the best. For example, an extremely low blood glucose level may require taking a test a short time later or at another time altogether.

When I was a staff member at a diabetes camp, I was in charge of carrying around the blood glucose meter to help check and treat low blood glucose at the Friday night dances. Dancing is exercise that makes blood glucose go low. I was amazed at how many kids came over to me to check, thinking that their blood glucose was low and they needed a snack. Only about half would actually be low. Some had perceived low blood glucose because their blood glucose did drop from all the exercise of dancing, but it didn't drop too low. I couldn't help wondering if the others were experiencing excitement or anxiety or even a place to escape from the social pressures. The kids were concerned—as all kids might be—with being picked to dance or hoping to be liked by someone special. It is easy, even for adults, to interpret uncomfortable feelings as the start of low blood glucose. Testing is a good way to start checking things out.

A teacher should applaud himself if he is not overwhelmed, and respect himself and get help, if he is. You can be a wonderful ally in managing the disease.

Teacher to child: You see the 11-year-old child with diabetes from your class eating several big helpings of cake in the cafeteria. You do one of the following:

1. Snatch it from her hand. (Admittedly, this is a tempting solution. It is, however, aggressive and humiliating to the child, and it only works in the short term.)
2. Assume she knows what she is doing and say nothing to avoid a confrontation. (This slightly resembles positive reframing but leans heavily toward passive cowardice. It might not be the best time to speak to her about it.)
3. Tell the mother later. (This places you in a tattletale position that breaks the trust between you and the child.)
4. Say to the child later, in private, "I'll bet you are glad the eating guidelines have changed, and there are no restrictions on sweets. Is it still hard not to eat too much when you are around friends? Could I be of help to you when you are at school, either before you make choices that aren't so good or after, figuring our how to be honest with your mom and balance your blood sugars?" **(Assertive empathy, normalizing behavior,** and **assertive questioning** means you are an ally and can begin problem solving.) If it were an ongoing pattern, you might say, "Let me sit down with you and your mother, and I'll support you while you tell her how hard it is not to eat extra in school. She needs to know, and I would like it to be from you."

Teacher to parent: The mother of a child with diabetes calls you several times a week. You can't return her calls until the end of the day, and when you do, she is always angry. You do one of the following:

1. Postpone calling her even though you know it makes her angrier. (Procrastinating only makes it worse for both of you).
2. Call her back with anger, telling her she is demanding, and really letting her have it. (This makes a great fantasy but is not professional behavior. It is aggressive and not empathetic. By putting off telling her what you are able to do to help, you increase your own anger and hurt yourself, too.)
3. Let her know you do not make phone calls until the end of the day and explain what it feels like to always have her angry with you, especially because you are putting in a lot of effort to learn about diabetes. (Excellent assertive sharing of your feelings; even if she doesn't change, you can feel relieved that you have taken care of your feelings.)
4. Say, "You know I have been working with the school nurse and am reading up on diabetes. Are you having a problem trusting that I know and will call you if I see a problem or a pattern emerging?" (**Assertive questioning** leads to getting more information that may explain the necessity of the calls from the parents' point of view.)

BABY-SITTERS

To me, a hero is someone who does something they don't have to. Choosing to learn about diabetes signifies something about your good character, willing to go the extra mile to help a family when you could have simply worked for another family.

You can feel especially good that you are giving a family a much-needed break. You don't have to cause yourself undue stress, however. Your decisions don't have to be perfect. Just do the best you can and keep learning. You will have to be more like a parent, rather than a friend on the issues around food and mealtimes. Remember the word *normal*. Make your authority decisions the same way you would for a child who does not have diabetes.

Susan was an excellent baby-sitter, unafraid to learn about diabetes. She was happy to spend time with Tommy, a 10-year old who has had diabetes for 3 years. One afternoon, after they had finished rigorously skating, Tommy had a low blood sugar that did not respond to the usual box of juice. Susan knew he needed more. She remembered about the glucagon injection but had never given it before, so she decided to call 911. It was, of course, a good decision in this case, but Susan felt she had failed him. Like a well-meaning parent, she second guessed all she should have done to prevent the whole thing or how else she might have handled it. She felt terrible about herself, sure that everyone was disappointed in her.

Susan made many excuses about being busy and unable to continue baby-sitting. The parents felt guilty they had not done a good enough job teaching Susan and thought she was angry with them and the responsibility of Tommy. Susan and Tommy were both heartbroken about not seeing each other. Finally, seeing how unhappy Tommy was at losing his "big sister," Tommy's parents got up the nerve to approach Susan and ask her to forgive them. "Forgive you?" she cried. "I'm the one who's ashamed. How could you ever trust me again?"

It was such a relief for them all to understand how each of them had misinterpreted that day's events. The parents knew they would have felt the same way about having to give a glucagon shot if they had never done it. And when the parents went to find the glucagon, they realized the prescription was out of date. In fact, Susan had done the right thing. They all went together to the nurse educator to have a review session and iron out their fears and self-doubt. In diabetes, low blood glucose happens. And so does panicking or calling 911, followed by a return to normal blood glucose, leading to stories that may seem funny in retrospect.

So, baby-sitters, just continue to learn about diabetes, be open to new ways of doing things, and apply the same good judgment that you do with every child. Most important, enjoy that child, who just happens to have diabetes.

The Medical Family

We've come a long way baby. From assuming that social or emotional factors in a patient's life have nothing to do with the outcome of a physical disease, to employing alternative medicine strategies for coping with medical problems. Our focus and way of doing things is changing. The most important change for you is the idea of having a team of medical professionals to help you with all the aspects of good diabetes care. The next most important thing to realize is that you, the patient, are the captain of the team. Your health care providers don't do things to you, we do them with you!

WHAT IS A HEALTH CARE TEAM?

In 1976, I was an inexperienced social worker in a busy county hospital. There was a special patient, a young black teenager named Benny who had frequent bouts of DKA. I was bothered by how sick he was when he came in and how quickly he turned into a delightful kid with a huge appetite. "DKA just happens," the medical staff said, "so move on to your next case."

I contacted Dr. Jay Skyler, and he began to answer my questions and help with the case. Ultimately, the explanation, but not the solution, became clear. Benny stopped taking his insulin shots whenever he felt overwhelmed and was actually clinically depressed. He lived with an aging grandmother who loved him but had limited resources or energy for him. He needed many things besides insulin. Dr. Skyler and I were determined to help him get those things and stay healthy and out of the hospital. It was nice to have a professional partner in this. And that is where the idea of working on a team was born for me, and for Benny.

People with diabetes need a couple of families—the one they are born with, the one they create, and their medical team. It is the medical team that gives the necessary ongoing support to you and your other family. The team can keep you, your family, and each other from burning out. No one has to carry the burden of care alone, and everyone is interested in doing their professional best for you. They share an interest in you and your family and support you in developing your problem-solving skills.

YOUR POSITION

You are the captain of your health care team. You're the leader, we're your helpers. Although you have to put it into action, developing a plan that works for you is a cooperative effort. You can learn from your medical team to evaluate each situation and make decisions about your care. You should be actively and self-confidently involved during and in-between office visits. With a chronic disease, it's not "take 2 aspirins and call me in the morning." Now, when you think you've had a crisis, your physician might start problem solving by asking you first for your assessment of what went on and your treatment plan, reinforcing the idea that you are the expert on you.

THE MENTAL HEALTH COMPONENT OF THE TEAM

Psychologically, the health care team helps you identify emotions, strengthen your self-confidence, and thus be able to participate in good self-care. They help you make healthy behavior changes.

You may not realize how intimidating, at times, you and your feelings can be to the health care team. You don't have to wear a white coat to make people nervous. Take a moment to empathize with how difficult it is for your health-care professional to respond to your feelings or answer questions in a way that always makes you feel good. They are only human, too. They can get as frustrated as you do when your blood glucose levels don't behave the way you want them to.

There is a mutual frustration with unmet expectations. Sometimes the confrontations between you can feel like the team is accusing you of not telling the truth—sometimes accurately, sometimes not—such as when records differ from lab results. Don't ever feel that you should lie about your practices or actual blood glucose results. Unconditional love from the medical team means that they are there for you, regardless of how well you are doing. They need honest feedback if they are to assist you in problem solving and getting the best care for yourself.

AN UNUSUAL RELATIONSHIP

Dr. Ronald Goldberg is unique in his perspective and relationship skills. When necessary, he tells some of his patients that he is not giving up on them, but if they want to continue working with him, they have to trust his advice and participate in psychotherapy to really be able to take care of their diabetes. Doctors can set conditions for how they want to work with you while they still care unconditionally about you. It is like tough love. This might feel like rejection or unfair limits to you. But it is a sign of how much your provider cares about you.

The practice of chronic health care requires an unusual relationship between doctor-patient-family. Change does not happen solely by giving information. Patients often know what to do but still can't get started. Many times they will begin to do things at first to please the doctor or their parents. That is a satisfactory beginning. The next step is to continue taking good care of yourself because it is something you want to do. Becoming healthy is a process with natural ups and downs.

TEAM APPROACH

Another benefit of the team approach is that it offers many ways to understand a problem. This became apparent to me in one of the first cases I was involved in, at the end rather than the beginning of the problem-solving process.

Jane was an 8-year-old with diabetes, who was delightful and very shy. She continually had low blood glucose before lunchtime, even to the point of passing out. The family and the team were worried and tense. They tried various regimens of insulin. They tried different meal plans. The staff knocked themselves out with ingenious problem solving. The problem continued. Why on earth couldn't they prevent her from having low blood glucose?

There were no obvious problems. Stalling for time because I was not sure what direction to take, I asked Jane where she would eat her midmorning snack. She honestly answered, "I don't eat it. I don't like to get up in front of everyone." There were incredible sighs from all around. This was a case of nonadherence for a clear reason by a very nice child who had not been directly asked some questions, except accidentally by me. Often children and adults don't have the courage to volunteer information because they think the doctor won't approve or they may not be aware that the information is important. Medical people, too, can get caught up in being kind rather than curious and nonjudgmental.

CHANGES IN THE HEALTH CARE SYSTEM

Some research suggests that it is not the length of time of your appointment but the kind of communication that is the strongest factor in getting you to try to come closer to treatment goals. This becomes very apparent to professionals in practice. More and more medical schools are acknowledging this in their curriculums. Once involved in practice, physicians may include a mental health person on their team for service to the patients dealing with chronic disease and other members of the team.

DOING YOUR PART

Here are some practice exercises for checking whether you know how to interact in healthy ways with your medical team members. Healthy, direct communication from

You have type 2 diabetes and have dreaded going to the doctor because you have gained 5 pounds and have no blood glucose records to show him. You force yourself to keep the appointment anyway, despite fearing a confrontation.

Provider: It looks like you have done none of the things that we talked about. I don't know what I can do for you today.

Patient: Don't answer right away. Take time to become aware of your feelings. You recognize that you feel miffed, embarrassed, scolded, and ashamed. You want to say, "Forget this, I am never coming back here." You also begin to daydream about what you will eat as soon as you leave the office to cope with your pain and embarrassment. However, you cannot afford to get lost in righteous indignation about how insensitive he is. Move on to the goal you hold in common: how to live with diabetes.

Breathe. Take a moment to keep your impulsive reaction in check by looking at the situation from your doctor's point of view. How do you look from over there? Are you giving him all the information he needs to understand your point of view? He is frustrated by not being able to help you and perhaps, the annoyance is not directed only at you. Breathe again. You can feel more relaxed when you realize that your behavior can affect his feelings, too. The main issue here is how you can get the help you need to take care of your diabetes. Having processed these feelings, you can be clear about your goals and ready to respond.
Now, you can make any of the following responses:

1. Actually, I am proud of myself for not canceling this appointment even though I did not do what we had planned. That feels like a positive change to me. It means I am not avoiding my responsibilities. It also means that I believe I can work with you. **(positive)** (Not getting distracted by his point, but sticking to your own.)

2. You might be right. Working with you is probably not enough. I need lots of support and ongoing education. Do you have a team of people you can set me up with? **(nondefensive agreement** and **assertive questioning)**
3. Making these changes is very hard to do. I wonder if you might put yourself in my shoes and have more patience with me? **(nondefensive** and **assertive request)**
4. I can hear the frustration you have in working with me. **(assertive empathy)** Does that give you some understanding of how I feel about working with my diabetes? **(assertive request** for empathy)

you will affect the response you receive from them. Note the skills that both parties need. You can use these ideas as a jumping-off point for discussion with your medical team. [The conversations contain exaggerations to make certain points and are not meant to offend any person or profession.]

You cannot afford to let your emotions take over in this situation. The point is for you to stay healthy. If you choose a different route, such as blowing up or stomping out, you might "win the battle, but lose the war."

THINKING ABOUT THE MEDICAL TEAM'S POINT OF VIEW

Having compassion for the medical family actually helps you.

Diabetes increases your responsibilities, interactions, and feelings, so you and your medical team need specific skills to make it all flow more smoothly. The skills involved are the ones we have spoken of all along, the same skills that families need.

COMMUNICATION SKILLS

1. **explore:** ask questions without judgment
2. **positive reframing:** repeat the information in a positive light
3. **empathy:** take the other person's point of view
4. **normalize:** say how what seems negative is normal
5. **nondefense:** just listen, don't focus on responding
6. **problem solve:** define the issue, come up with solutions, and test them
7. **positive confrontation:** be direct without criticism or negativity
8. **clarify values:** prioritize the things that are important to you

SITUATIONS TO SHARE

The following are situations that often come up. Keep in mind that sometimes health professionals may react to the tone of irritation in your voice or to what feels like rejection of their medical advice. These examples are written in a playful spirit, to help you and your

MEDICAL TEAM

Your patient with type 2 diabetes has gained weight.
You say:

1. I give up. Would you like half of my sandwich? (Tone of voice is important, or this is going too far. He can't really give up. On the other hand, it is kind of funny and makes a point).
2. I give up. It is your life. (Hostile. This is poor role modeling. You don't want your patient to be a quitter, too. Anyway, you care about what happens. Underneath your reaction are feelings of frustration, discomfort, and sadness.)

3. You need a shrink. (Perhaps you need some help figuring out how to help this patient? Consulting with mental health professionals on difficult cases or issues can be refreshing. The need for therapy is not negative, not failure. If you say it in a negative manner, your patients are not as likely to go.)
4. What are your thoughts and plans about the 10-pound weight gain? **(support** and **exploration)**

This is nonjudgmental, will get you information that you need, and get your patient to be clear about his responsibility in this.

Your patient with type 2 diabetes has maintained his weight rather than lost weight.
You say:
1. It looks like you can't help yourself. (Uh, oh. Frustration is leading to an aggressive put-down and not helping you focus on the good parts—he returned for the appointment and maintained his weight.)
2. It looks like I can't help you. (It helps no one for you to feel like your patient ignored you or that you are ineffective. People are complex. Motivating through guilt doesn't last long, either.)
3. What would motivate *you* to start losing weight? **(exploration** and **problem solving)** (Great, get the person involved! Make an individualized plan together.)
4. It is impressive that you are maintaining and not gaining weight. **(positive reframing)** (Accent what has been accomplished. Small goals count.)

Your patient says, "I will lose weight when you do."
You say:
1. How rude.(Are your feelings hurt? Your patient's hostility is misguided. It is the burden of losing weight, not you or your advice that he minds. Pain is underneath the biting words. Try to listen to patients, so when the air clears, you'll have something helpful from the message.)

continued

2. It's your life. (Your answer shows that you're offended and angry, emotionally about to abandon this patient. Nobody wins.)
3. Well, I don't have diabetes. (He has a point, and you know it. Being overweight, you are at risk too. At any rate, good role models are worth a thousand lectures. This patient may be good for your health.)
4. It must be hard to have to do what others around you do not. **(empathy)** How can I help you with your success? **(nondefensive)** (Good job, you stayed on track for his issue.)

The mother of your 15-year-old patient feels overwhelmed.
You say:

1. Don't worry, be happy. (Good advice for a song, and a well-meaning attempt to comfort. I would add, "I wonder if you would consider a support group or teaming up with another parent of a child the same age?")
2. No one controls diabetes during adolescence. (You mean to be positive, but this is inaccurate and discouraging to both of you. Low expectations don't motivate.)
3. Go to a psychologist for family therapy and parenting skills. (Good advice, but depending on how it is said, the parents may feel it is just one more burden or something else for which they will be blamed.)
4. Many of my patients experience difficulties during adolescence. Diabetes does add difficulty to the normal growing pains. I am referring you to our team psychologist, as I do many of my patients, for support and ideas in communication. **(normalizing,** supportive, **problem solving)**

Your patient has a high hemoglobin A_{1c} (average blood glucose reading) of 12%. Surprisingly, his records show all normal blood glucose levels.
As a physician, you:

1. Knock your head against the wall. (Hopefully you are wearing a helmet.)
2. Scold your lab technicians. (Pass the buck; make it a mistake of the lab.)

3. Ignore it. (Comfortable, tempting, but this is passive and not kind at all if you're trying to avoid the confrontation that would save this patient from having to lie and the danger of poor blood glucose control.)
4. Acknowledge how difficult diabetes is **(empathy)** and address the discrepancy directly. **(supportive confrontation)**

Your patient says, "This diet is just too hard to follow."
You say:
1. Obviously, you gained 5 pounds. (aggressive)
2. Well, try again. (passive) (Probably won't work because you don't yet understand why it wasn't effective the first time.)
3. I appreciate that. Diabetes is demanding. **(empathy)** What parts are you able to follow? **(accent strength)** What parts are you having difficulty with? **(problem solving)** What are you willing to do differently? **(values clarification)**

Your patient says, "My wife and kids and your office staff eat everything in front of me."
You say:
1. You have to have self-control. It is *your* diabetes. (Defensive and moralistic, even if it is true.)
2. I can hear how frustrating it is to be exposed to all these temptations. **(empathy)**
3. Do you think you could let your family know that you want to bring home a healthy lifestyle? **(positive reframing)**
4. What would be hard about telling them what help you need? **(support** and **exploration)**

health care professionals develop the ability to laugh at yourselves in the high-pressure but rewarding team management of diabetes. Feel free to share them, or use them to help you recognize communication traps and difficult situations that make you feel bad or cause you to offend someone else. Role playing your medical team's position may give you a new perspective on your own behavior.

It pays for all of us to think (sometimes, quite a lot) before we speak, so we are sure to speak to the real issues. Remember, hostility is not honest. It is just a spontaneous reaction to hurt, frustration, disappointment, or anger.

AVOIDING STEREOTYPES

The following are some issues that may derail you or your medical team. These stereotypes, like most prejudices, can be overcome with awareness, patience, and information.

The elderly and diabetes. An elderly person is someone who is 10 years older than you! Not many people identify with being elderly, but there is definitely a stereotype. Aging is not sickness, but there may be losses in physical strength and abilities (taste, hearing, vision) that may affect your desire or ability to manage diabetes. The team must help motivate and educate you about good diabetes care and teach you coping skills. Let them know if you have economic concerns or problems with friends or family helping you. Also alert your team to any symptoms of depression, anxiety, or substance abuse that might be impairing your health.

Likewise, diabetes must be taken seriously as an illness. It is not a natural process that comes with aging. Your health beliefs, such as how serious you think the illness is, what consequences you think it will cause, or even if you believe the treatment will have an impact, will determine how you handle diabetes. Your physicians and other team members need to clarify their own beliefs and prejudicial ideas, such as elderly people can't handle diabetes, why bother them, or they are too set in their ways. No matter what your age, you are a worthwhile, whole person. For your part, ask lots of questions, and let your doctor know that you are willing to do more than he thinks you can.

You can learn what to do. Research shows that elderly patients who were taught to do home blood glucose monitoring prospered in their care. Doing something so you don't feel helpless is a blessing. Of course, you feel well when you get closer to normal blood glucose, and you're more likely to keep on taking care of yourself.

I remember my mother being devastated when her physician told her not to bother watching her cholesterol. He said, "At your age, it doesn't matter anymore." She felt unimportant and powerless and began to think that her actions would have no effect on her health. In the end, he appreciated her feelings and pointed out that he was only trying to make her life easier.

The health care team must help you set realistic goals that fit you and your family.

Catherine, age 70, lived alone all her life, never married, enjoyed a satisfactory career, and has been obese all her adult life. She has had diabetes for 10 years and done nothing to care for her health. When she came to our team, she began to check and record her blood glucose for the first time. With this watchfulness and some increased medications, her blood glucose came close to normal, but her weight did not change. The team was constantly after her about losing weight. Each week she came in and was labeled "unsuccessful."

At one appointment, Catherine got furious, saying that we were beginning to remind her of her mother for whom she had never been "good enough." There was always one more thing to do before she would really be okay. Catherine said that she was pleased with her progress, and if we weren't going to be too, she'd go somewhere else. She taught us a good lesson. In retrospect, we realized that we all should have been pleased. For the first time in 10 years, she was controlling her blood glucose and maintaining her weight. What happened to small, realistic, mutually agreed on goals and positively reframing behavior?

Adolescence. Here are a few special words for a very interesting period. Not only families but also the medical team respond strongly to people this age. Pay attention to your team's *countertransference*—the feelings aroused in the professional about the patient or his situation. Countertransference can occur with any patient, but adolescents have a particular flair for igniting it. The physician, depending on his or her perspective, life experience, or particular place in the life cycle (does s/he have a teenager?) may bond and side with either the adolescent or one or both of the parents. Beware. The medical team cannot afford to alienate either the teenager or the parents.

Not feeling successful with the adolescent can make the health care provider impatient or angry. The indifference that adolescents often show, masking many other feelings, can be alienating or intimidating.

We have to be accepting of the *feelings* of the adolescent, if not always their *choices*. Observing the situation without judgment but with honesty and compassion can work in these situations.

When the patient is a health care professional. When a health care professional gets diabetes, s/he needs the same instruction and repetition and still may not do what is suggested. (Remember that knowledge alone is not enough to make people change.) Adherence problems usually stem from emotions, not knowledge. Professionals may be reluctant to ask for guidance because they are ashamed they do not know what is expected of them. But unless diabetes is their specialty, they are no more likely to know all they should than someone who isn't a health care professional. Even when health professionals have knowledge, just like other patients, they may not take care of themselves.

Women. In the past, medical research was done primarily on men, so we don't know whether there are significant differences in diseases in men and women. But we're catching up. We do know that women, from adolescence on, have higher rates of depression than men. The risk is increased again by having diabetes. It is thought that the diagnosis of depression may be missed in 75% of cases. This is important because depression is directly linked with poor glucose control and subsequent complications of diabetes. It can lead to weight gain, smoking, lack of exercise, and generally not following through on diabetes management. It can, in essence, change a woman's personality.

A health care team needs to be sensitive to the special issues that a woman's cycles bring. We must acknowledge that hormones and menstruation can cause high blood glucose levels, food cravings, or the phenomenon of insulin resistance. Your team should cover preconception counseling (beginning at an early age to keep mother and baby healthy), pregnancy, and the relationship between complications and sexuality. Menopause may bring with it temporarily disturbing physical and mental symptoms and the hormone swings can disturb glucose control, too. Through all the stages of a woman's life, support groups and one-on-one meetings with other women with diabetes can be very helpful.

Obesity. *Obese* is a medical term signifying a condition of being 25% over ideal body weight. Patients don't like the word, and the medical team may inaccurately assume that obese people have character flaws rather than a complex medical problem. Our society does discriminate against obese people, sometimes causing them to dislike themselves.

Recent weight-loss guidelines suggest setting small goals in weight loss rather than trying to achieve ideal body weight (whatever that is). Sometimes those guidelines are not satisfying to patients. Let your health care team assure you that small goals work better and are longer lasting. In fact, losing just 15 pounds can improve your blood glucose control and lower high blood pressure. You can feel satisfied with and proud of these attainable goals and then add your own. Don't connect your self-worth to physical size. The emphasis should be on healthy eating rather than dieting, on variety and nutrition and not food restrictions, enjoyable exercise, emotional support, and getting rid of everyone's prejudices on weight discrimination.

Multicultural issues. Aspects of culture—such as traditional roles of men and women, foods, cooking techniques, or exercise choices—will affect how well you adhere to medical advice. Your medical team needs to be aware of your cultural background and your point of view. The culture you were raised in affects the way you see the world. Your world view is connected to your diabetes care in many ways. *How do you think about* ***time?*** *Do you worry about the present or future? How does your family see* ***developmental tasks?*** *Do they believe you are separate and independent? Do they regard you or the family as the patient? Which cultural* ***rituals*** *need to be included in your diabetes care plan to make you feel comfortable? Does your medical team have knowledge of your* ***customs?*** Looking you in the eye means cooperation to the medical team but it signifies disrespect in some cultures. *What family* ***roles and gender*** *expectations are you dealing with, or what does being a man or a woman with disease mean to your family? Does a man need his physician to be an authority?* Your **religious** orientation can strongly affect your diabetes management. *Do you believe diabetes or complications are your destiny or it's all in God's hands?*

Medical teams need to be aware of cultural differences because, without this sensitivity, they may be impatient with what seems like a lack of motivation. However, in becoming culturally sensitive, we must be careful not to stereotype people because there are so many variations among ethnic populations, and individual differences within groups. For example, European American families expect separate identities for individuals within families and encourage independence. This is different from the interdependence that is important in many Hispanic and African-American families. A tightly knit extended family is valued throughout life and the medical team may need to involve more of the family in appointments. In a Hispanic family, a grandmother bringing the child to the appointment does not imply that the mother and father are not interested. Not letting a child go to diabetes camp or do his own insulin injections are also aspects that the medical team might call overprotection. It is important to understand what feels right for a particular family and work with them.

It helps when patients have to make the claims of their culture clear to the medical team. (There is, after all, a medical culture with definite doctor nurse roles and practices.) Perhaps when you have discussed your cultural values with your health care provider, and you feel that they are respected, the medical team can start to help clarify conflicts you and your family have been struggling with instead of adding to them.

It's way out of proportion, but diabetes and some complications of diabetes are more common in African Americans, Hispanic Americans, American Indians, and Pacific Islanders. It is important for all of us to try to understand the factors involved: heredity, environment, social and economic stresses, attitudes toward health goals or providers and style of care, and the stress of discrimination upon health. Dr. Alan Delameter documented that excess stresses on the children of some minority families, as perceived by the mothers, is related to poorer blood glucose control. We cannot underestimate the impact of living with these chronic stresses, which can suppress the immune system and make people more likely to get sick.

Marsha was a young black child who had been shuttled around in foster care because of an abusive mother and absentee father. In the middle of all this, she was diagnosed with diabetes. In an odd way, it may have been the one thing that saved her. She came to our medical family, and now, at age 30, she tells us that we were the one constant support for her as she grew up. She was exposed to support, feeling loved and cared for, getting the attention she needed both medically and emotionally, and mentors for new and different goals for herself.

The medical team was careful not to "pathologize" Marsha's acting-out behavior of ignoring her diabetes. We had to account for the stresses in her life—poverty, abuse, foster care, and contacts with racism in her daily life and in the foster care system. Our medical priorities were different from her preoccupations and cultural issues. Buying fresh vegetables and testing strips to use four times a day seemed way out of line, at first. In the beginning, our medical team was just another system of mostly white people who were intruding on her life, making demands on her, giving instruction, and implying that she needed to do a better job than she was doing. While we could never make up for the lack of strong and steady attachments in her life, we did make a difference by providing her with new or on-going relationships that taught her competence, self respect, and discipline.

In ethnic or immigrant families, there is a phenomenon known as *acculturative stress*. This is the conflict between parents and children over the children accepting cultural values different from their parents' native values. It can also refer to the individuals who feel they belong in neither culture. Members of the family have one foot in this country and the other foot in the country of origin. These individuals and their families are not in agreement about which culture is in charge—the new one represented by the medical establishment or the one they have known most of their lives. They are not comfortable in the new culture, but they don't have the security of the former one. Taking the best of both worlds, and allowing each to be part of the identity in a rich biculturalism is helpful.

The dangers in adolescence may also be seen as acculturative stress. The child is caught in the middle of wanting to be the child who is cared for but a teenager in a new world where he doesn't want to be any different from his friends. As a group, teenagers have to deal with pressures to smoke, drink, be rebellious, take risks, and be spontaneous, but those behaviors do not mesh well with the organized daily diabetes control that their families expect.

Iliana was the very Americanized Cuban-American wife of Jose who has had diabetes since he was 12. They were both 32 years old and had been married for 5 years. Iliana was incensed that her mother-in-law was constantly interfering in her adult son's health. In her American-culture mode, she wanted a complete separation from the mother's direction and control. Whereas these issues overlap with personal and interpersonal dynamics, there was clearly a cultural value from the mother's generation that welcomed her into her son's health care. At another place and time, her involvement would have been expected. To reduce the stress of being caught in the middle, Jose asked the medical team to help. The team first had to work out its own conflicts that came from their differing viewpoints on gender, family member, and professional roles. They were then able to enter this arena with insight and leadership—smoothing the relationship between Jose's wife and mother, and bringing in Jose's father, too—and improve Jose's health.

Psychological insulin resistance or nonadherence? When physicians realize that it is time to suggest insulin to their patients, they hesitate for many reasons:

- fear of upsetting the patient
- possible future hypoglycemic crises

- increased time required for teaching
- hope that the patient will lose enough weight or increase exercise and not need insulin

When a person with type 2 diabetes is told that s/he needs insulin to get normal blood glucose levels, s/he resists feeling that s/he has "failed," or is truly sick. S/he hates shots and feels that now s/he'll become a slave to diabetes. S/he, too, wants a chance to try again. Calling this "psychological insulin resistance" or predictable procrastination recognizes that the patient and the professional both are hesitant to make this change and are putting off insulin therapy—leaving the blood glucose out of control longer than necessary.

A high percentage of people with type 2 diabetes will eventually need more than diet, exercise, and oral hypoglycemic medication to reach the goal of near-normal blood glucose levels. If you need insulin to help you reach your blood glucose goals, do not think of yourself as failing, even if you are overweight. Your body needs insulin, that's all. And keeping your blood glucose levels near normal, no matter how you do it, helps you prevent or slow down any complications from diabetes.

Complications: Putting the Accent on Prevention

This is a difficult chapter to read, as well as to write. I know some of you will avoid reading it because the subject matter is frightening. It is about things that you hope never become part of your life. However, to gain some peace of mind, face your fears and support yourself with information and stories. The ideas raised here may just scratch the surface of the feelings and issues you may be facing. You need to be the expert, because you live with diabetes everyday. In this attempt to give order to something that does not unfold neatly in real life, remember that many complications can be prevented and that getting one does not mean that you will get any others.

It may be helpful to look at your original emotional response to the diagnosis of diabetes. See how far you have come since then and how you've learned to cope in new ways. You have also learned something about your strengths and abilities, haven't you?

Then think about what the diagnosis of a complication means to you. What are your first thoughts (self-talk) likely to be? *I knew it would happen, I give up. What should I do with my life now? How will my spouse take this? What about health insurance? Is taking care of myself now still worth the trouble?* It can be devastating to be told that you have traces of protein in your urine (proteinuria), or changes in your eyes (retinopathy), or damage to nerves in your feet (neuropathy). Complications call up an entirely new but, as we've said, revisited challenge. Personal reactions are complex and varied, but you are thrown back to the feelings you had at the initial diagnosis of diabetes—anxiety, fear, guilt, and rage.

You can't just worry about the past or fear the future; you must focus on the present and what this challenge means for you. This meaning will affect how you take care of yourself. Once you figure out your personal meaning, you will have to be patient while the meaning takes shape for your spouse, kids, and work. With all these feelings and having to come up with a plan of action, it makes sense to jump in bed with the blanket pulled over your head, for a little while. Hopefully, after awhile, you can get up and deal aggressively and positively with taking care of your health.

Even if you do develop a complication, you can and must live a full life. My friend and colleague Gary Kleiman has lived with diabetes for 38 years, and only 12 of those years have not included complications. He is to be admired for his humor, hard work, and ability to enjoy life. He says that he accepted the responsibility for something he did not choose to happen with a protective layer of defiance or anger that helped him keep his balance. In the early years, he did not like being different because of his diabetes, but now he sees that diabetes is part of what developed his creativity and ability to see things differently and in a new way.

At 18 years old, when he was beginning to lose his vision, he was frightened and angry and could not understand how an artist and a tennis player could possibly live with being blind. Remarkable how things can change. More than 25 years later with a kidney transplant and legally blind, Gary hits a mean tennis ball, is passionate about his work, is a wonderful sculptor, and loves his terrific wife and two healthy children.

FIRST STOP IS PREVENTION

The good news is that complications can be prevented, or when they do develop, they can be stopped and sometimes even reversed. The DCCT and the Kumamoto study (of people with type 2 diabetes) taught us a lot. **Bringing your blood glucose levels near to normal and keeping them there has an astounding effect on complications.** Add regular checkups to catch retinopathy or foot ulcers early and you will be in the best possible shape. Research shows that 85% of limb loss and 90% of blindness is preventable by these techniques.

Now, improving your blood glucose control may not be easy for you nor is it inexpensive. You will need to check your blood glucose levels more often and to learn more ways to balance food, exercise, and medication to meet your target levels. Get help from your health care provider or nurse educator to be sure that you are testing correctly and that you know what adjustments to make when you get your blood glucose reading. You need to be physically active so all systems of your body work better. And you may have other health concerns. You need normal levels of blood pressure and blood fats such as cholesterol, and if you smoke, get help and give it up. These measures will help you avoid the heart and blood vessel (cardiovascular) problems and kidney disease that diabetes puts you at risk of developing.

There are things to do beyond attempting good blood glucose control to keep you healthy that some people neglect. Sometimes it is due to limited health insurance, finances, transportation, or knowledge. For example, did you know that laser treatments can significantly reduce blindness but only half of people who have diabetes get a yearly eye examination? You need to see specialists who are trained to discover any diabetes-related problems early.

Did you know that high blood pressure is hard on your heart, blood vessels, and kidneys? Have you spoken with your health care provider about the ways you can bring your blood pressure down without using drugs, such as exercise, changing your diet, and stress management techniques? Did you know that losing 15 pounds helps lower your blood pressure and improve your blood glucose control? Do you know what foods to eat to improve your blood fats levels?

Did you know that comparatively more people with diabetes smoke than people who do not have diabetes? And that it takes them longer to quit? Did you know that smoking multiplies your risks for diabetes complications? To quit smoking you can join a group, get hypnosis, try acupuncture, or take medications or use nicotine replacements, such as gum, patches, or nasal spray and antidepressant medication recently approved by the FDA. It has been suggested that yoga helps, because the deep breathing is much like the deep breathing that a smoker does—only healthier. But first you have to decide to quit.

You may do that through conversations with family, friends, and medical people. Quitting smoking is difficult because it is an addictive behavior, but you also have to work through the emotional concerns over stopping, such as feared weight gain, fear of withdrawal symptoms, and social anxiety. What will you do when you're not smoking? Make that decision to quit.

THE FIRST COMPLICATION: DAMAGED SELF-ESTEEM

An unrecognized complication of diabetes is the effect that having this chronic disease has on your emotions and self-esteem. This includes living in a preoccupied, self-conscious, or anxious state.

Diabetes can make you feel different beyond the extra required tasks and lifestyle changes. Help yourself and your family members make sure that feeling different does not equal feeling inferior or less than whole. Minimize the negative feelings and create an attitude that you can handle special challenges in a heroic way and more often think about yourself as special or unique. Anything with a positive slant will do.

The issue of lower self-esteem can affect everything from job and social issues to marriage and parenting, and certainly will be a problem in the event of physical complications occurring. A hardy self-image has got to come from deep inside.

I have seen people avoid activities, fearing that others would "see" their diabetes, such as having a low blood glucose reaction with too much physical activity. People wearing insulin pumps have told me that they felt their only choices were not to go swimming at all at the beach with their families or to go and feel self-conscious. What about going and enjoying it? It is emotionally hazardous to avoid things that are pleasures or to feel that you need to overcompensate for who you are. Diabetes is hard enough without adopting a point of view that interferes with you having a good time. You are who you are. Everyone is different in some way.

Gary reminded me that he went through years of enduring difficult comments, other people's unkind judgments or annoying questions. The negative tone can be like a thorn in your side that accumulates over the years. Gary explained to me, "I got it to stop, but that doesn't mean it didn't happen." It made me sad I couldn't have followed him around when he was a kid, keeping him out of emotional harm's way. I know this is the same feeling your family and friends have.

You can't stop other people from saying things. All you can stop is the way you take what is said. How you feel about comments and how you respond is what you can control. Thick skin helps. Verbally attacking them may make you feel better for a moment, but you might get better results by assuming that they mean no harm. They're not knowledgeable. You have an opportunity to help them learn, if you feel like it. If you are calm and wise, they are more likely to learn how to be that way, too. Often the best offense is no defense.

FEAR

Fear of complications can keep you from doing the things that will keep you healthy, ruling your mood and your actions. It can keep you from learning what you need to do or from asking for help from those who can help you.

Focusing on fear of what you might lose can keep you from enjoying what you have in the present and limit what you achieve in the future. Taking care of yourself out of fear is not as long lasting as finding positive goals, such as feeling good from being in control today.

Lenny, a college sophomore with diabetes since he was 15, made this concern come alive for me. I had not seen him since he had gone off to college. Early one Sunday morning, I received a phone call from Lenny from his college dorm room. "Can you talk?" he whispered. "It finally happened." Caught up in his sense of secrecy, I whispered back, acknowledging that I was alone and was ready to listen. "It finally happened, I am impotent." Lenny proceeded to tell me the whole sequence of events. It started off with "We went drinking..." and ended up with his attempt to have sex with someone he had met at a bar.

I was so glad that Lenny had called. It would have been terrible for him to continue thinking his assessment of the situation was accurate. His fear of getting complications had overridden his knowledge about diabetes and perhaps had caused some of his careless behavior. His fear had made him miss the point that overindulging in alcohol—possibly resulting in low blood glucose—and unprotected sex with an unknown partner were the probable causes of his being unable to maintain an erection.

As he told me the story, he realized these points for himself. Then he felt relieved and understood that he had some thinking to do about how he wanted to live his life, and how not to live in fear. He asked for an appointment with me and his endocrinologist on spring break, 2 weeks away. Now that he was a young adult thinking about his future, he realized that his values and goals needed to be readdressed. Meanwhile, he was going to take a look at his drinking habits to determine whether he was having a problem.

When complications do actually occur, you need a supportive and informative relationship with your friends, family, and medical team. People can operate out of misconceptions. At these times, they need input from their medical team, just as Lenny did. Communication was a positive first step in dealing with his fears and concrete problems.

NO SUPPORT

Loneliness seems to be connected to giving up. I observed this in a support group I lead for patients with diabetes who have experienced below-the-knee amputations.

John was a 58-year-old single gentleman who had known he had diabetes since he was 50, but probably had it much longer. The diabetes was picked up when he complained about impotency to his physician. He was depressed and disinterested in his own care. He avoided a social life, giving up all relationships with women, concerned that no one would be interested in a man who was impotent.

People are in better health when they have companions. John's avoidance of all personal contact reinforced his depression that also kept him from facing his diabetes care. He was uninterested in nutrition or exercise guidelines. In line with this thinking, he did not pay any attention to the details of neuropathy in his feet. He was overwhelmed with having to face the loss of part of his leg. For the first time, he was facing it with a supportive group of other patients and interested health professionals.

We were very intent on knocking John over the head until he agreed to antidepressant medications, rehabilitation services, and participation in intensive follow-up. He agreed to involving his local church, a neighbor, and a niece in his ongoing care. It was a difficult time in John's life. He cried in the group because of his losses and in response to being cared about. Meeting with others disturbed him because he could not escape from the reality of his situation. Giving up seemed easier. Reaching for and taking help was new to him, and it felt awkward. He promised he would try to battle against giving in to low expectations for his life. We hoped he would continue to let us be an ongoing part of his life.

When you develop complications, family, friends, and medical people interested in your healing can give you contact, support, motivation, accurate information, and hope—practical and spiritual. However, the family is also feeling increased anxiety and depression. Ironically, at the time that you may be most needy, other people, including your medical family, are sometimes not there for you. It is difficult to hear another person's despair, anger, anguish, or panic. And we all need to overcome this and be present for the other person.

GRIEF

A person who has lost part of his or her vision must take time to mourn for the sighted person s/he once was. The healing will come from letting go of what was. The entire family needs to grieve, but parents, spouses, and children can set aside their own grief in the beginning to be a support for the person with diabetes. Take turns.

Dr. Naomi Remen, in her book *Kitchen Table Wisdom*, talks about how it took her a long time as a physician to realize that for patients to heal emotionally and physically, they needed compassion as much or more than they needed medical expertise.

ONE COMPLICATION, NOT NECESSARILY ALL

In diabetes, a complication can often stop progressing abruptly, and go no further. Research from the DCCT, for example, suggested that tight control not only reduced the complication of neuropathy from occurring by 69% but could also decrease its progression once you have it by 57%.

Getting tight control must be accomplished slowly, with the help of a medical team, so that any frustrations or problems can be understood. Good control can temporarily bring low blood glucose reactions, weight gain, or even some neuropathy pain, so you might misinterpret it as not being worth it. Having guidance along the way can help you keep on track.

The beginning of a complication does not signal the beginning of other problems. Please make sure you and your family are aware of that. This information is significant for encouraging yourself to stay in tight control to prevent worsening of that complication and to keep other complications from occurring. Of course, the initial response to a complication for individuals and their families is a period of being sad or angry or hopeless. Later, this stance must be traded in for good diabetes management.

Edward was part of a support group that had been meeting together for several years. He is a 43-year-old man with type 1 diabetes who had started a course of laser treatments on one eye. One evening in the group, he was crying and speak-

ing of his devastation and hopelessness surrounding the procedure and his fears of laser treatment. He said he'd rather die than be unable to see. The rest of the group, who had also shared many personal feelings and ideas over the years and thought they knew each other well, was listening intently, everyone's eyes wet with sorrow for him. Members responded with genuine empathy and understanding for all the feelings Ed was having.

Later, two other participants, Nora and Cindy, each shared the experiences they had gone through 10 and 15 years before with laser treatments. They had been in the group for 6 months, and no one had known about their experiences. It was not that they forgot to tell the group, it was just not something they thought about much in the frightened way that Ed was feeling. Nora and Cindy were amazed at themselves. Time and distance had helped them accommodate the worry they thought they never would give up. They both remembered how much emotional pain they were in and how lonely they felt at the time of their surgeries, not knowing anyone else who was going through it.

They described that the hardest part for each of them had been waiting for their eyes to stabilize—6 months for Cindy and 1½ years for Nora. What seemed most difficult for both of them was not knowing how much vision loss there would be. The unknown frightened them the most. They remembered being impossible to deal with as they were going through this. They were impressed by how long ago all that seemed. Edward intently absorbed their words and began to find some solace.

BEYOND SELF-BLAME

Nora explained how she had given up taking care of herself for a while in the midst of her problems with her eyes. She realized through therapy that she had blamed herself for it happening and felt she did not deserve anything better. In the beginning, she resisted efforts in therapy to ease the sense of guilt so that she could try to take care of herself and enjoy the things that were okay in her life. In her answer to the why me? question, she found guilt easier to deal with than helplessness. She had no control over getting diabetes, and she was desperately trying to feel that she could direct what happened to her next.

Her guilt made her feel powerful in a strange way because it meant that she could control her life, even if it was poorly. Obviously, some people with diabetes do not take care of themselves, and complications don't happen to them. But self-blame and guilt can be useful if it enables you to say, "I caused it, and now I will fix it."

When the vision problem started, she told her doctor that she would kill herself if she ever lost her vision. The doctor tried to be understanding of her feelings. He insisted she see the team of professionals, including the ophthalmologist, psychologist, and psychiatrist that he had cultivated to help his patients with diabetes.

Nora started taking care of herself again when she moved past the original grief. A psychologist helped her stop taking her anger out on herself. Forgiving herself was going to lead to forgiving diabetes, too.

She could then turn to thoughts about what she could control, the stabilization of her diabetes to prevent any worsening of her eyes or development of other complications.

A FULL LIFE

Nora continued her story. She had changes in her vision. She was filled with frustration and rage. She was impatient with everyone. It seemed to her that people who didn't have diabetes took so many details in their lives for granted. She was stuck, wondering when or whether her eyes would stabilize. Other people could run out at night to pick up a movie without worrying about blurred vision. They could read the newspaper everyday, not thinking about their ability to read. Life did not seem fair, once again. Wasn't diabetes enough?

Nora would change from her angry feelings quickly to her guilty ones. She had not taken care of herself, had deliberately acted out her feelings, and soothed herself using food for much of her life. The therapist she worked with helped her understand that she had an eating disorder. She was getting rid of the excess calories by letting her blood glucose run high and losing the calories in her urine. Then she was frustrated by knowing she had another chronic illness, the eating disorder, to contend with. Gradually she began to feel a sense of relief and understanding. She sobbed and sobbed over all the sadness and fear she had never been able to face or share.

After Nora finished telling her story, people in the group who had known her for several years were surprised that she had been through so much and had not needed to talk about the vision problems anymore. It was reassuring to them that if Nora could get over all that, then they could live with less fear, too, realizing that whatever losses might ever occur to them, they could get through it.

NOT A STATISTIC

How do you live with statistics in the first place? What do you do with thoughts of which complications will happen to you? If you read that 30% of patients with diabetes will be affected by kidney disease, that means that 70% will not be. Why not see yourself in that 70%, especially if you take care of yourself? Can you make a deal with yourself not to live with worry and fear over your head but to live in healthy denial with healthy practices?

PURPOSE AND PASSION, IN SPITE OF IT ALL

Franklin Delano Roosevelt showed us how powerful one can be despite a disability. Sometimes people with diabetes complications will put off doing the things they can actually do out of self-consciousness or fear. They worry that others will ask too much or that they might not feel well, get too tired, or have to leave in the middle of a dinner. In a reversal of an old saying, Dr. Remen suggests that "anything worth doing is worth doing half-assed." Her point being that people ought not to stop themselves from enjoying their lives because of imperfection, worry, embarrassment, or the fear they won't complete things.

Is it worth it? Yes, it is always worth making an effort to act positively on your life and to enjoy it. At times you will have to make a determined effort to push yourself, and while there, to focus on the enjoyable part. You can prepare speeches to make to yourself for encouragement. Prepared statements can be delivered to those around you when you need to interrupt your activities.

If you don't feel well, you get up in the middle of dinner and say, "This has been fabulous. I loved being here this long. You are all wonderful company. I must go home now. Shall we plan dinner again next week?" If you don't drive in the dark, rather than not go to dinner at all, tell your friends or hostess you will leave before dessert. (And before cleanup. There are some advantages.)

There is evidence that psychiatric symptoms such as anxiety and depression often increase in people who are in pain, for example, from neuropathy. Pain is aggravated in people who are not involved in something meaningful, such as work, volunteering, hobbies, sports, or interactions with other people. More than ever, even if there is discomfort, interacting is part of the healing process.

DEPRESSION

There are several causes of depression for people with diabetes. The simplest can be the fact of having a chronic disease. Other causes are the biological connection to out-of-control blood glucose, an inherited tendency for depression, the unending tedium of taking care of diabetes, and certainly complications developing. Studies suggest there are two times as many women as men who are depressed, but many less men seek out treatment, feeling that they are expected to be strong and silent. (See *I Don't Want to Talk About It: Overcoming the Secret Legacy of Male Depression* by Terrence Real.)

Clinical depression must not go undetected or untreated. Improving your state of mind allows you to begin to learn the coping skills and self-care tasks necessary for good control of diabetes. Sometimes families don't know what to look for or what to do about depression. Othertimes people are aware there is a problem but decide they should fix it themselves, and won't rely on doctors, therapy, or medication. They don't realize that receiving help is the key to being able to accomplish health goals.

Antidepressant medications help patients see through the forest of depression to discover their natural coping skills—or at least open up a space to develop some. Part of recovery from depression is self-help:

- reading
- increasing activities
- challenging your negative thoughts
- learning to think positively and constructively
- helping others

SYMPTOMS OF DEPRESSION

If you have three or more of these symptoms, and they last for two or more weeks, it's time to get help. If you have the last symptom, seek help immediately.

- changes in sleeping patterns—too much sleep or insomnia
- changes in eating habits—weight gain or loss
- consistent feelings of sadness for more than 2 weeks
- feel tired all the time
- have difficulty concentrating
- feel nervous or anxious most of the time
- feel guilty or that you're a burden to others
- feel hopeless or that your life is worthless
- have thoughts of suicide

DEPRESSION AND SELF CARE

If you have type 2 diabetes and you need to lose weight to avoid the need for insulin, you should understand that the difficulty may be depression. Don't avoid treatment because you're ashamed or frustrated by the weight or because your pride says that you have to do it yourself. You can get wrapped up in your feelings of being different because of diabetes or depression, and you avoid interactions with family members and professionals on these issues. You may want to keep accepting a bad mood as just the way it is, blame others, be alone until it passes, or use food, alcohol, or drugs to give you a lift. These are self-help techniques that do not work. Timely professional treatment of depression, including maintenance treatment, helps keep the depression from getting worse or returning.

Poor attitudes of self-care and depression are linked to obesity, failure to follow diabetes-care plans, increased smoking, alcohol abuse, and limited physical activity. These symptoms are often undiagnosed by families or medical professionals and often don't receive the attention they need. A further interesting connection is that patients with diabetes who smoke have more symptoms of depression than those who don't smoke. This suggests that smoking may be a coping mechanism for handling depression. Smoking is too damaging for people with diabetes and makes their chances of developing several serious complications much more likely.

Sometimes depression in diabetes is overlooked by medical people because of the lack of training, the expectation that you will be feeling badly, other symptoms are masking it, or appointment times are not long enough.

OBESITY

There is a serious link between obesity and type 2 diabetes—60–90% of people with type 2 are overweight. Obesity is also linked to a host of other medical complications. Approximately one-third of all Americans fall into the category of obesity, a jump of 25% in the last generation.

The treatment for obesity (and type 2 diabetes) is weight loss, especially modest weight loss (10–15 pounds to begin with) and maintaining that to make an impact on blood glucose control. Adding some physical activity can work wonders too. This is a positive change from the all-or-nothing attitude about weight loss that physicians and patients associate with frustration, failure, and regaining weight. Research has shown that overweight people who are physically fit are healthier than thin people who do not exercise. Exercising does not have to result in weight loss to make you healthier.

Other treatments for obesity are to learn healthy eating habits and to monitor blood glucose and learn how to balance food, exercise, and medication. Behavioral therapy, which includes learning what and when you eat, goal setting, and reinforcement, with a professional will help you be even more successful over the long term. Small changes are important in improving exercise and food habits. Obesity is a chronic illness in itself that can be managed with a long-term program and care (understanding not judgment) from a supportive health care team with counseling skills and patience.

Weight loss, eating fiber-rich foods (vegetables, fruits, whole grains), and exercise also help prevent type 2 diabetes for those who are at risk with family history.

EATING DISORDERS

An eating disorder can be a complication of diabetes and can cause other complications. Be conscious, not worried. Most people with diabetes do not develop eating disorders. The necessary focus on food and weight in diabetes can make you question whether you have a problem. You probably don't. However, if you never think that you are thin enough, no matter what your weight is, or you deliberately change your insulin or medication to lose weight, you do have a problem. Letting blood glucose levels run high all the time means that a change in routine or other health status could put you at risk for a life-threatening condition that can lead to coma and death. Certainly, chronic high blood glucose puts you at risk for complications. Get professional help.

In diabetes, food can become a preoccupying aspect of your life, and other people—family and medical team—are necessarily overinvolved in your personal habits. The diagnosis can make you feel helpless at first and cause you to try to bring a sense of control over your life with the use of food. This is the one thing that children and adolescents have control over.

Sometimes professionals or families can miss the diagnosis of eating disorders even as we are complimenting patients on their weight loss or low blood glucose, not realizing that they accomplish this at the expense of good diabetes care. I was concerned about one young girl and educated her mother about the issue, but the mother was still more focused on how happy she was that her daughter was thin. She told me the secret of her daughter's success had been in drinking lots of water. Only the third elevated glycosylated hemoglobin test convinced her that the drinking resulted from the thirst of high blood glucose levels. Her own desire to be thin and to have a daughter like her blocked her from acting on what we already knew. Prevention strategies and speedy discovery are of the utmost importance. Eating disorders are more difficult to treat when they are entrenched as patterns in an individual's life.

Eating disorders appear as a preoccupation with dieting and thinness. While food (eating it, getting rid of it, or avoiding it), body image, shame, and secrecy appear to be the main issues, the underlying feelings encompass powerlessness, depression, anxiety, loneliness, anger, and all-or-nothing and perfectionist thinking. (See chapter 6 on parents.) The disorder finds resolution in the external solution—food, diet, thinness—rather than the internal solution—regulation of emotions.

Anorexia. Anorexia is characterized by a drive for thinness; pursuing weight loss or, in the case of children, refusing normal weight gain; an exceptional fear of becoming fat, regardless of being very underweight; a disturbed body image; and lack of menstrual periods in females or loss of sexual interest or potency in males. The way to get thin is to restrict food through fasting, dieting, and exercising. Mood disturbances are made worse by the state of semi-starvation. Losing weight may initially be an attempt to achieve a sense of control and feel good about oneself. It changes into an obsessional preoccupation with weight and denying oneself food.

Bulimia. In bulimia, individuals are preoccupied by their weight but have periods of giving in to their desire to overeat and then, regretful, try to take control through purging. The binge-eating periods include an amount much larger than others would eat, sometimes many thousands of calories. During the binges, individuals have an out-of-control feeling that they cannot stop eating. The binges are followed by restricting food or excessive exercise or various purging methods. The additional danger in diabetes is purging by intentionally omitting or reducing an insulin dose for the purpose of getting rid of the calories. (An action that can lead to ketoacidosis and coma.) This is more difficult to detect than anorexia because individuals have near normal body weight. They are more aware than people with anorexia that their behaviors are different and unhealthy, and they are more interested in receiving treatment.

Binge eating. Binge eating is a common problem, suggested to affect 20% of people who are obese. Binge eaters are not so concerned with weight loss, and the binges are not followed by the purge cycle found in bulimia. Generally the individual does three or more of the following: eat rapidly, eat when not hungry, eat until overly full, eat alone because of shame over the amount, and feel distress over their eating, which leads to feeling depressed and guilty. They do not emphasize weight control, and they gain more weight. Episodes of binge eating usually occur at least 2 days a week for more than 6 months.

Lisa Schwarz's research showed the association of binge eating with weight dissatisfaction, poor adherence to diabetes care, and levels of depression.

The patients who need help with this are often older, there are more males in this group, and there is an equal number of African Americans and Caucasian Americans. A mental health professional can help with underlying depression or mood disorders and appropriate medication.

Insulin manipulation. Another sort of eating problem (but not a clinical condition) is the occasional poor usage of food or insulin and a negative preoccupation with one's body. This affects a significant portion of the population with diabetes. Insulin manipulation is thought to be related to fears of weight gain or concern with hypoglycemia. Research by Dr. Polonsky suggests that 31% of individuals omit insulin at certain times, but 8% do it frequently, risking severe consequences.

DIAGNOSIS OF EATING DISORDERS

With diabetes and eating disorders, there are elevated hemoglobin levels, hypoglycemia from purging or food restriction, and episodes of ketoacidosis. Eating disorders can seriously damage the health of people with diabetes. To treat them successfully may require education, therapy—individual, marital, and group—and antidepressant and antianxiety medications. Of course, exercise and nutritional counseling are vital.

With the diagnosis of an eating disorder, families may have to wrestle with self-doubt, guilt, blame, resentment, and anger at each other as well as the person with the disorder.

With the help of professionals, families can adjust to new guidelines and structure that is good for the prevention of eating disorders as well. They will need to learn to

- balance privacy and separateness
- allow conflict
- deemphasize appearance so self-worth is not dependent on weight
- focus on feelings not food
- make mealtimes pleasant
- stay away from controlling or scolding about food behaviors
- discuss what situations are uncomfortable (for example, eating out in restaurants)
- continue to do the things that are satisfying and pleasurable

The most important of these may be focusing on feelings, not food. As we've said, diabetes brings up powerful feelings. If you do not have healthy ways to acknowledge and live with those feelings, you are likely to use food as an unhealthy way to cope.

COMPLICATIONS CHANGE THINGS

Living with complications puts more pressures on you and your family. Physical and emotional effects of complications can contribute to changes in financial status; the roles you handle at home or at work; the amount of energy you have for work, social life, and sex; mobility with walking or driving; sleep patterns; kinds of entertainment such as reading or sports; and sometimes even independence itself. Aging is not a complication, but it does affect diabetes, emotions, and physiological changes.

Dr. Robert Shuman touches on the intimate physical and psychological adaptations of his own experience with multiple sclerosis in *The Psychology of Chronic Illness: The Healing Work of Patients, Therapists, and Families*. He says that when there are concrete physical and emotional losses, individuals have to make shifts in how they perceive themselves. Your values need to make a shift, too. You begin to emphasize integrity, relationships, kindness, intellect, and goodness over or as much as the more traditional values of physical appearance, social roles, and money. Making room for the self-image to thrive amongst all these losses is difficult. Sometimes patients see the losses as personal failure or the physical problems as embarrassing and can be reluctant to share the problems even with their physicians, which prevents the conditions from being diagnosed and treated.

MARRIAGE

With increased stress on you come additional pressures on your marriage. If there were already problems, the extra stress (more than the complication itself) creates havoc. Your partner who doesn't have diabetes may have to pick up duties that cannot be accomplished in the old way. When there is a concrete physical loss such as a change in vision, you will have an increased physical and emotional dependency on your partner that may be difficult for both of you to accept.

The most difficult part for you may be getting the people around you to hear your fears and confront your realities with you. People—including the medical team—are often afraid of another person's pain and may either avoid it or try to prematurely cheer you up. Sometimes you may feel unlovable or guilty about the changes and cannot figure out how your spouse or you are going to live with the complication without anger and sadness. This is where your responsibility lies. Work through the anger and sadness to get to a better emotional place. It is the chronic, not the initial attitude about your complication, that will drive people away or bring them close. Keep the lines of communication open with your family, enjoy each day as it comes, and avoid negative expectations of what the future holds for you.

When I married my husband, Jim, he had type 2 diabetes and had already gone through bypass surgery. I was intimidated by his health status on paper but experienced him as a strong, virile, athletic man. I remembered that when my mother married my stepfather, George (she was 59 and he was 70), he too had many medical problems and didn't look good on paper. Rumblings went on in the family over the wisdom of their marriage. They defied the worry of the well-meaning skeptics through intense affection and love for each other and led a honeymoon of a life for the next 17 years. They were good mentors for how love has the opportunity to bypass medical problems. Jim and I are doing the same thing.

Several years after we were married, Jim had a second bypass surgery. We had much to learn about feeling okay about the return of his physical strength. The delight of stage two in our adjustment was realizing that there was life after sex after bypass surgery. I had not expressed any anger for the first year after bypass because I was concerned about how it would affect him. Stage three in our adjustment brought us the knowledge that there was life after arguing after bypass surgery.

The one advantage for our marriage, anyone's marriage, is that we both appreciate his vulnerability and want to keep our stress levels down. With this in mind, we approach any of our conflicts with total honesty but with an emphasis on tolerance, kindness, and self-control over anger. The irony is that, because of his complications, we consciously treat each other respectfully, as people do in the beginning of courtships. Our lives are more enriched, not less, through dealing with all his illnesses. At some point, complications need to be seen as an opportunity to be connected and personal. Don't just slip back into the resentment or responsibility that it also brings to both partners.

EXERCISE

Exercise will help improve your emotions and your physical health. It's the best thing to do for complications. Unfortunately, various complications of diabetes can interfere with your usual routine. You may have to change to swimming rather than walking on a treadmill if you lose sensation in your feet, or discontinue heavy weight lifting and change to swimming or walking if you develop proliferative diabetic retinopathy. You may have to test more often if you have hypoglycemic unawareness. Finding the appropriate amount or type of exercise based on the complication is essential.

If you stop exercising, what do you expect your family to do? They will miss your physical and emotional well-being. Have you stopped prematurely out of fear? Have you discussed any concerns or problems with your family or health care provider? There are solutions to ease your fears. And ways to overcome the obstacles. If you've been overweight or never exercised in your life, you may be self-conscious about your coordination, appearance, or lack of experience and fitness. Just begin with a level that you can handle. Take a walk. If you think you'd enjoy other sports or activities, get instruction on how to do them correctly and practice until you feel comfortable doing them. Make activity part of your regular day. More than anything else you do, physical activity makes you feel better physically, mentally, and emotionally.

STRESS

Stress management training can help. Some exciting research by Dr. James Blumenthal of Duke University has shown that heart patients who involve themselves in formal stress management training can cut their risk of heart attacks or the need for surgery by 74% compared to patients under routine medical care. This tremendous difference was accomplished through a group intervention program that simply had weekly 1½-hour sessions that highlighted knowledge, support, and skills in reducing stress.

PHILOSOPHY

Gary Kleiman and I have worked together and been friends for 20 years. He is a model for winning his personal battle with diabetes. Gary has lived with complications for 26 years, so far. He lives a full life. He has never just accepted his fate but fought for and has taken advantage of progress in diabetes care. At the time of his kidney transplant in 1983, he wrote an inspirational book titled *No Time to Lose*. I keep encouraging him to write his next book, *More Time Than I Thought*.

> **SERENITY PRAYER**
>
> God grant me the serenity to accept the things I cannot change,
>
> the courage to change the things I can,
>
> and the wisdom to know the difference.

When all is said and done, complications, and the fear of them, can bring monumental change and are frightening for the whole family. Please think through these concerns, do lots of communicating, and get the help of others, so you can make good decisions about your life, live life to the fullest, and have a sense of inner peace along the way.

The Diabetes Prevention Program (DPP) is the nation's largest-ever research study to determine whether type 2 diabetes can be prevented or delayed. Screening at one of the 25 medical centers across the United States is free. If you are interested, call toll free at 1-888-377-5646 for more information. The program is sponsored by the National Institute of Diabetes and Digestive and Kidney Diseases, which is part of the National Institutes of Health. If someone in your family has type 1 diabetes, others in your family may be at risk of developing it. Two clinical trials, sponsored by the National Institutes of Health, are in progress. To find out more, call the national Coordinating Center at 1-800-HALT-DM-1 (1-800-425-8361).

Spirituality: Finding the Meaning of Diabetes

We all know we are going to die; the important question is how are we going to live? As a culture, we seem to be on a quest for meaning. People are flocking to psychologists, spiritual teachers, classes, books, horoscopes, and all the new (or ancient) methods for expanding spirituality. There is a renewed interest in religion. The pursuit to find meaning seems to grow out of a need to balance overwhelming stresses from outside and bring equilibrium to the turmoil inside us. A spiritual search offers us an opportunity to step away from the everyday aspects of our lives and to get new perspectives. Spirituality is where we find good values to commit to, a way to connect with and give to others, and peace for ourselves.

This chapter is a brief exploration of spiritual ideas—both mainstream and alternative—as food for thought and discussion. For example, people who worship regularly are nearly twice as likely to quit smoking and one third more likely to start an exercise program.

You do have a choice. Your mind creates your experience of happiness or suffering. Look at what you're thinking. *What gives your life meaning? What makes you feel connected and comfortable? How do you handle your responsibilities—of diabetes, work, school, friendship, parenting? What parts of life do you treasure and enjoy? How do you maintain balance and quality in your life?* The answers lie partly in your personal concept of spirituality, the core of your energy and your values. Your behaviors are based on your personal view of the world.

Besides the strain of coping with busy modern life, people with diabetes and their families also try to make sense out of *why this, why now, why me, why my family? Is there a God? What have I done to deserve this? Why does a good person suffer? How can I face my life? What is actually important?* These thoughts flood your and your family's minds as you adjust to the diagnosis of diabetes and attempt to deal with its daily demands. In addition, you have to make peace with the fear of complications.

Spirituality helps you make sense of your life and health. Finding meaning in your life leads to better emotional and physical health. When you are curious about spiritual matters, you are more likely to follow your diabetes care plan, too. It is true wisdom not to limit your happiness and health to the physical body.

WHAT CAN YOU LEARN FROM ILLNESS?

On Friday, I was reviewing which patients were coming in for the week-long hospital stay on Sunday night. Sylvia was 22 and blind from diabetes—unusual for someone so young. I anguished over a few things. I was overwhelmed and depressed by a young person having to go through such a terrible thing. I had heard many patients tell me in the past that they would rather die than live with blindness. What did I have to offer her? If I was having trouble anticipating interacting with her, I wondered how the young kids coming for the week-long course would feel. I worried that they would be too upset to learn or commit to renewed efforts in their own care.

My mistake came from ignorance and anxiety. I had not anticipated Sylvia, only her complication. She was funny, outspoken, positive, smart, and ambitious before she became blind. She remained that way afterwards. She told us we were lucky to meet her now, a year after it had happened, because she went through a terrible year and so did everyone around her. Sylvia was enlightening and inspiring to all of us. She said that she had always enjoyed life and could not give that up, in spite of any obstacles. She believed in God, a loving God, and she assumed He did not want her to stop enjoying life. She laughed, saying that she hoped blindness was the last hurdle, or she'd have to change her name to Job, from one of the oldest stories in the Bible.

Sylvia decided to move forward positively well before her family did. She trained as a professional massage therapist, using her heightened sensitivity to touch and her desire to enjoy and be close to people. She found organizations handling services for the blind and while doing research there, she met and fell in love with a man who had also been using the services for the blind.

During that week, the rest of the group had their fears aroused, seeing a young person with such a serious complication. But her optimism and spirituality helped each of them make peace with these fears and put the energy of worry into taking better care of themselves. Sylvia was more committed than ever to keeping her spiritual nature strong, not only for her sake but because it was powerful in other people's lives, too.

Sylvia's story reminded all of us of what we can control—*attitude* and *efforts*. Calling herself Job reminded us of the story that challenges us to understand why terrible things happen to loving, caring people. Job was a religious, successful, and loving family man who, despite his goodness, was struck by dreadful events, each one worse than the one before. Stripped of his family, wealth, and health, he kept his faith and believed in life. He chose to focus on being glad about all the joys he had once had and to be pleased with whatever he had left. Job's religious and spiritual beliefs gave him the power to endure and love his life.

FAITH AND ILLNESS

Rabbi Harold Kushner wrote *When Bad Things Happen to Good People* to tell stories of struggle and acceptance. It has been a source of comfort for people like himself who have chronic illness or are related to someone who does. He suggests that nature, not God, causes disease. The importance of this perspective is that it allows you to see illness not as failure but as part of the natural law. It is not your punishment or a judgment cast on you.

There are indications that spirituality not only makes you feel better but makes you physically better, too. Mind and body are intertwined and won't stay in neatly labeled boxes for proper medical treatment. The body heals itself and there are more factors that influence healing than prescription medicines or a hospital stay. Healing does not depend solely on the body. The spirit must be involved, too.

PART OF EACH DAY

The busy pace of our lives, loss of extended families, and an overinvolvement in the material world have left us hungry for our natural spiritual nature. Meditation, learning to focus, and paying attention to the present moment are ways to feel better and connected. These practices are powerful tools for sorting through spiritual confusion.

We can begin each day with an effort to slow down and notice our spiritual being. We might find ourselves using secular or nonreligious ways to do this, such as a morning run, a 12-step program, or yoga. To follow a more traditional religious path for spiritual expression each day, you might recite a morning prayer to welcome the day or attend a church service before work.

THE SPIRITUAL DIRECTION

Lisa Schwarz, a strong, resilient person and excellent diabetes nurse educator who's had diabetes for 28 years, is—despite or because of her experiences with diabetes complications—a very spiritual person. I have watched in amazement and deep respect as she has refused to allow bitterness, anger, or cynicism to darken her point of view. She remains focused in herself and generous to others with knowledge and support. In the 20 years I have known her, she has reminded me of what she learns from listening to others and to her own body. Diabetes is first a psychosocial and spiritual condition and, second, a medical condition.

With this in mind, Lisa suggests that we need to know more details about patients and their families. *Do you have a healthy balance among life, work, relationships, and diabetes that enables you to feel energetic, at peace, and lov-*

ing? About the diabetes, she hopes that you are in tune with yourself. *How do you feel about your diabetes the majority of the time? Are you doing a good job and learning more or are you feeling depressed and defeated? Did you stop checking your blood glucose? Are you not interested in diabetes education? Do you eat high-fat foods? Can you get support from family or friends?* If the answers that come to mind are more negative than positive—and possibly in many areas of your life at the same time—this indicates a crisis in the spiritual realm. Negativity diminishes your sense of peace.

ATTITUDE, ATTITUDE, ATTITUDE

Expecting a positive outcome and following self-care routines is the action that puts the worry to rest. Forgiving life for the test you've been given and accepting diabetes comes next. Then you can catch and remove any negatives as you go along.

As you can see, the spiritual can include but is not necessarily limited to a religious perspective. One difference between spirituality and religion is that spirituality is more universal, with no fixed dogma or practices. Joan Borysenko, a psychologist *(Healing the Body, Mending the Mind)* is a tremendous resource in exploring the mind-body-spirit connection and describes our generation as experiencing a "crisis of meaning and values in life, and a lack of spiritual optimism." She considers the spiritual side of her patients with the dignity it deserves in medical circles.

Dr. Jean Shinoda Bolen *(Close to the Bone; Life-Threatening Illness and the Search for Meaning)* suggests "illness is a soul event that is often ignored." This is particularly true in the diagnosis of diabetes, which necessitates so much learning and doing. Her concept is that healing must occur for the mind, the body, and the spirit. Healing can occur in the soul, even if the physical body doesn't make it to the same level.

Donald, a 62-year-old man with type 2 diabetes, impressed me with his ability to make peace with what was happening to his body. Neuropathy had made it difficult for him to walk without using a cane. Other patients in the same situation felt understandably bitter and, rather than use a cane, they took risks with falling or chose to eliminate activities outside their homes, sealing the lid on the depression that came with the complication. Donald had similar feelings, but he reported to me how he turned them around after taking a long-planned vacation trip with his wife.

He started out markedly aware of having a disability. By the end of the trip, he saw the cane as getting him preferential treatment. He boarded airplanes first, people opened doors for him, and they gave him smiles of respect and encouragement (he chose not to read the smiles as pity). Somehow the cane had succeeded in elevating his status as a person, not just a body. The responses of others had reminded him that his life had to be more for him than the bitterness he was legitimately feeling. He began to hold his head up high and smile at everyone who would look his way and let his energy in. He felt people admiring him for his good nature and courage. With his openness, they seemed willing to respond and even cater to him. He viewed the cane as a powerful extension of himself and dropped the sense of disability that had been becoming his self-image. Don said that maybe he let this spiritual perspective in so easily because he did not think he was deal-

ing with a permanent disability. He was looking forward to the neuropathy getting better but he wasn't sure if he was going to give up the cane.

When life doesn't seem fair or when we cannot make sense of what is happening through normal logic, we can turn to the spiritual.

I had a patient who had been diagnosed with a series of illnesses. Each time she suffered through them, doing what she had to do but never fully taking care of herself or prioritizing her needs, at least in addition to those of her husband and children. She never seemed to learn anything from the illness, never broke stride with her repressed anger, depression, and her selfless ways. When she was diagnosed with diabetes, she cried out, "Enough. Why are things still happening to me? Life is unfair. I hate my life." Indeed life had not been fair to her. After validating much of her sorrow, together we focused on trying to find some meaning and purpose.

What made diabetes different from the other illnesses was that if she did not stop and take care of herself, she would suffer immediately. She would either have low blood glucose from not having time to eat because she was trying to please her boss, or she would have high blood glucose from grabbing high-calorie junk food to avoid going low. Either way, she would be tired and unable to concentrate and frustrated with the effect on her blood glucose levels.

Despite the uncomfortable feelings and much education and emphasis on communication skills, she had not been able to change her behaviors. She was able to take action only when she adopted a new perspective that diabetes was given to her because she needed to learn a lesson that she had not yet learned from all her other health problems. *To stay well, she would have to tend to herself.* When she found the spiritual connection, she took time to make sense out of her life and her diabetes. She had a sense of peacefulness that she had not felt in years and began to focus on what she could control and enjoy.

LOVE IS HEALING

Deepak Chopra, a physician and communicator with many helpful books, suggests that the spiritual is who you are, not what you do or how much material wealth you have accumulated. In the case of diabetes, the spiritual is not what your body is doing but how you are doing. He, along with many others, says that nurturing the soul is accomplished by concentrating on tolerance, compassion, courage, love, wisdom, and generosity to others. The Pope, on his trip to Cuba in 1998, urged "Whether you are believers or not, accept the call to be virtuous. This means being strong within, having a big heart...being courageous in freedom, generous in love, invincible in hope." These are the virtues that actually relieve our suffering.

Dr. Dean Ornish has done a great deal of work on reversing heart disease in his patients through diet, exercise, and stress management. In his book *Love and Survival,* he says that giving and receiving love has healing power because of the connection and meaning it adds to our lives.

HOW DO WE GET THERE?

Dr. Jean Shinoda Bolen says, "For a soul to be heard, the mind must be still." When you procrastinate on self-care tasks, is your mind full of criticisms, self-doubts, and worry? You can replace the worries with a conscious spirituality, achieved through a process of slowing down. You can slow down through breathing, prayer, meditation, yoga, chanting, music, mantras, affirmations, guided imagery, mindfulness, visualizations, friendships, reading others' stories, and helping others. With these activities bringing peace and quiet to your insides, you can outwardly practice living a joyful life. Any of these processes is helpful. They help you clear a path to look at what you genuinely value, who is really important to you, and what you really want to be doing.

Meditation. There are many ways to meditate, such as repeating prayers, watching a candle or a spot on the wall, doing yoga, saying a mantra, listening to music, chanting, or simply focusing on your breath. Concentrating on your own breathing is the simplest and most natural way, and you can do it anywhere and at any time. Meditation settles the mind and releases energy throughout the body. Herbert Benson and Jon Kabat-Zinn have written books about meditation that are helpful for people with chronic health problems.

The main skill in breathing meditation is simply paying attention to the process. It is best to sit in a com-

Self: This meditation feels weird. Besides, I really don't have time to do it now. I have too many things on my mind and stopping to do it will make me late.

Self to self: That's all true. **(nondefensive).** New things always feel strange, and you are busy. This is how you can stay busy and enjoy it and be healthy, all at the same time. Just try it. No more questions, just breathe. One, inhale. Two, exhale. You are doing great.

fortable position and breathe in through your nostrils. Observing your breathing and focusing on nothing else can be difficult. If your mind wanders, gently bring it back. To keep it focused, count the breaths in your mind. Count one as you inhale and two as you exhale, or some such rhythm. Breathing deeply and slowly is calming and invigorating. More oxygen moving from your lungs to your muscles gives you the feeling of being energized.

Learning to clear your mind comes with practice, just as learning to ride a bike does. Many thoughts will float through your mind, keeping you from focusing. Acknowledge the thoughts, let them float on by, and return your focus to your breathing. Do this gently and persistently, and your mind will settle down.

Yoga. This system of exercise is a wonderful way to tone the body through stretching and to calm it through breathing, relaxation, and meditation done all together. Aerobic exercise and strength training are more effective if you include stretching several times a week.

Mantras. Mantra literally means "something to lean the mind on." They can be nonsensical or meaningful phrases that are repeated over and over and over. You might repeat "Controlling diabetes is powerful," or "I am learning to love my body." Breathe as you say it and feel relaxation and positive energy fill your body. The meaning will become part of you.

Affirmations. These are positive statements or stories about you that you tell yourself. These do wonders to counteract the negative mantras that people use such as "I ruined the day by eating that" or "I can never finish one day perfectly." The statements you use can be built on truths that are specific to you. You might say "I am helping the insulin work as I quiet the stress" or "I exercise to help my husband with diabetes. I thank his diabetes for keeping me healthy. My husband thanks me." The affirmations are relaxing in themselves but also are great substitutes for the negative thoughts in your mind.

Guided imagery. When you are in a state of relaxation, guided imagery can tap your subconscious mind. To get into the relaxed state, imagine yourself going deeper and deeper into relaxation, perhaps as you picture yourself going down an escalator. Or imagine yourself in a quiet place such as a beach all your own. All the while, breathe slowly and deeply. Once in the relaxed state, you can let pictures come, for example, pictures of what your diabetes looks like. These will give you an awareness of what your feelings are about yourself and your diabetes.

You can also do guided imagery with a planned script that you can tape for yourself. "I am patting myself on the back as I go through another day. I've met 75% of my goals. I am smiling and entitled to be happy, in spite of my blood sugar number. I know how to get it down. I am excellent, not perfect." (See Carl Simonton's *Getting Well Again*, a book on using imagery with cancer that can be applied to diabetes). You can use imagery to make yourself feel okay about things in the past or to plan for the future by visualizing ahead of time what choices you want to make.

Imagine that you are on your way to a family dinner. In your mind, see yourself greeting your family. You have brought vegetable dishes with you for everyone to snack on. They even join you in a walk before dinner. At the table, you enjoy the meal (which fits into your meal plan) and the conversation.

After dinner, you are content and have well-controlled blood sugars. You feel disciplined, peaceful, and proud. In the living room, everyone is happily talking. You have no guilt, and the normal blood sugars promise you a good night's sleep.

Imagery prepares you for success. (Olympic athletes use it!) It can reinforce your goals and help you follow through on a positive plan.

Mindfulness. The attitude of mindfulness keeps you strongly focused and paying attention to the present moment, not preoccupied or concerned with the past or the future. It is about just "being," suspending judgment or fear. Mindfulness as an attitude is a particularly good antidote to fear of the future, perhaps the most difficult aspect of diabetes. Writer Alan Cohen *(The Dragon Doesn't Live Here Anymore)* says, "The present is the gift, that is why it is called the present."

Visualizations. These are stories translated into pictures in your mind. This might include picturing yourself smiling after checking your blood glucose, regardless of the outcome. You are happy because you are satisfied with where you are or pleased with where you are aiming to go with your next blood glucose check. Or, after giving your insulin injection, you close your eyes and see the insulin chugging along, happily making the rounds of delivering energy to your cells. Another visualization might be picturing your depression leaving your body like air slowly escaping from a tiny hole in a balloon.

Friendships. These give you a place to be your authentic self. Friendships are a significant part of finding and enjoying the spiritual side of life, through shared experiences and true intimacy.

The healing power of stories. Rabbi Simkha Weintraub of the New York Jewish Healing Center talked to me about biblical stories and Jewish folktales that help us find forgiveness, comfort, hope, guidance, direction, or optimism—all spiritual qualities. He shared an interesting and different interpretation from the story of Job by emphasizing how little help his friends were. They were invaluable in the beginning as they stood by him and grieved with him, but later, they discounted or blamed him, searched for meaning that could not be found, and tried to find what he had done wrong. Rabbi Weintraub suggested that what would have helped him, of course, was to "join him, to sit in silence, or to affirm his experience."

Rabbi Kushner's newest book, *How Good Do We Have To Be?*, says to get away from perfectionist interpretations of our own behavior and the behavior of other people. He cites a diminished self-love and love of others when there is imperfection, such as illness or the way people manage it. He observes that when children fight, they quickly get over it, valuing happiness over self-righteousness. He reminds us that only a forgiving nature, whether you are victim or aggressor, can keep us from having to relinquish our power to others.

The power of helping others. Victor Frankl, a holocaust survivor of Nazi Germany, was fascinated by what kept some men alive in the concentration camps *(Man's Search for Meaning)*. In a place where they had no choices, the survivors made a "soul choice" that no one could take away from them, choosing the attitude to take in response to the horror.

He chronicled several patterns in the camps: those who gave up (and died more quickly), those who were cruel to their peers and thought only of their own survival, and those who had a sense of loyalty to the group and took risks to help each other and share even little bits of bread. He found his own meaning by trying to assist others in coping. He and many others survived, physically and spiritually, by finding some personal significance even in this situation.

"It could have been worse," is a phrase I hear from many patients. I used to feel impatient, thinking that people were denying their sadness. Dr. David Gelernter, a survivor of the unibomber who lost a hand in the blast, surprised me when I heard him describe himself as lucky. His comments made me rethink things. He was truly in touch with what he had, not with what he lost in the bombing. He went on to criticize our victim culture. He made a clear spiritual choice to go on with his life in a positive way.

SPIRITUALITY: THE PROCESS AND THE GOAL

We can use prayer and stories and meditations as spiritual events we enjoy for themselves and as tools to change our health status.

It is through spiritual practice that we cultivate spiritual strength. Trying on new attitudes can be awkward, and we can flounder when we are practicing forgiveness, gratitude, or unconditional love. Our spirituality is a natural part of us that we overlook or don't give high priority. We have to train ourselves to notice experiences and be present in the moment.

FAITH HEALING

The 1971 White House Conference on Aging made an attempt to describe spirituality, but more serious study of how it relates to medicine was addressed in 1996 at a Harvard Medical School Conference on "Spirituality and Healing in Medicine." This conference invited an interdisciplinary and interfaith mix of participants and was led by Dr. Herbert Benson, a cardiologist who is known for his work on the "relaxation response" and its reduction of the effects of stress on physical health.

In 1975, Dr. Benson wrote a best-seller. In it he told how meditating or focusing on a single image could change heart rate, brain waves, and reduce the effect of stress hormones. His original work covered the practical medical reasons for meditating. His more recent work, *Timeless Healing*, suggests that spirituality and religion seem to trigger the same physiological process as meditation.

The role of the spiritual in medicine is profound. How else can we account for the placebo effect? When patients are given a pill that has no medicinal value, they improve because they believe in either the medicine or the doctor giving it. Though not religious, it is their faith or belief that heals them. What goes on between a patient with poorly controlled diabetes and the doctor during an office visit is not necessarily just an exchange of new facts and information. Sometimes it is the human connection and relationship and both of them believing in each other's capabilities that turns the patient around. A similar phenomenon is at work with effective management of pain, also sometimes an issue in diabetes. With a prescription that involves the spirit, relaxation along with medication or other techniques can help relieve the pain.

How can we account for the faith healing that various religions have recorded and the scientific studies of the prayer effect in Dr. Larry Dossey's research? *(Healing Words: The Power of Prayer and the Practice of Medicine)* Dr. Dossey documented that when patients were prayed for by others or prayed themselves, they lived longer and recovered faster from surgery, using less medication. An individual's answered prayer might be considered a placebo effect, but it appears to be more than that when the individuals who did not know that they were being prayed for from a distance had similar health benefits. It did not matter, in some of his detailed research, which religious group did the praying. Prayer by all faiths seemed to work.

Other researchers have shown evidence that people who have profound spiritual or religious beliefs, when compared to people without these beliefs, have fewer medical problems; have reduced rates of alcoholism, depression, and anxiety; recover more quickly when they have problems; and probably live longer. It appears that faith, not just the positive direction gained from religious or spiritual thoughts and activities, is independently responsible for positively affecting health.

Many researchers think the link between the spirit and health is the immune system, a concept know as psychoneuroimmunology (PNI). They document positive emotions and social connections having an impact on health. The power of social connectedness is shown through the finding that married people live longer than single or divorced people. Research on negative emotions also suggests that people with increased amounts of hostility are associated with higher mortality rates. Stressful experiences increase the levels of adrenaline and cortisol in the blood, suppressing the immune system. Controlled studies of laughter show its ability to reduce these levels and strengthen the immune system.

How can we account for spontaneous remissions and people who rebound from terminal illnesses? Dr. Bernie Siegel, a well known cancer specialist and author, classified patients as "exceptional" who fought their way to survival through challenges, emotional expression, and alternative or spiritual paths.

PHYSICAL EFFECTS

At this point, the medical community's interest in the spiritual process is directed at its impact on the body—that is, its ability to lower blood pressure or reduce pain. Meditation, taught by psychologists, is popular for its connection to physiological improvements, such as a lessening of stress and anxiety, issues that contribute to physical illnesses. This is a good place to start. You need no belief to get the benefits. It is just about doing it.

Because this is a practical book about techniques for dealing with diabetes, I have emphasized the pragmatic aspects of spirituality. I do not mean to shortchange anyone, and I believe that going to the soul level, regardless of its impact on the body, is important in and of itself. Dr. Shinoda says that when you get an illness, stop and focus on what needs to be better in your life on the body and the soul level. Dr. Lawrence LeShan, a medical psychologist, concludes from his research that "enhancing life, extends life." He found that people with a zest for life could more positively affect their own healing. He teaches and encourages meditation and taking time to focus on the present rather than being productive in some way.

INDIVIDUAL GROWTH

We are beginning to understand that creating a safe and spiritual place to nurture the soul will, in turn, nurture the body. Information is available, in books, conversations, religious services, support groups, and on the internet. If you begin to search, something will interest you, make sense to you, and resonate with or enhance your belief system. There are steps to go through to awaken your spirituality. Meanwhile, love yourself—as you are in the present moment—giving up shame and self-dislike, and take a moment to visualize who you would like to become.

> Seeking faith, they found hope.
> Hoping, they learned acceptance.
> Accepting, they discovered love.
> Loving, they lived or died.
> Loved
> Accepted
> Hopeful
> Fueled by faith—the path to wholeness and peace.
>
> *—Rabbi Gary A. Glickstein*

Putting Fun in the Family

This chapter is dedicated to reminding you that while diabetes is not fun, you are. Or at least you probably once were. And, of course, can be again. As small children, most of us were capable of being playful. Supposedly a preschooler laughs 400 times a day and an adult only 15. Now, don't start feeling guilty if you are underhumored. It is treatable.

LAUGHTER IS GOOD MEDICINE

Research has shown that the immune system is strengthened (as measured by blood tests) when research participants watched humorous videos. Laughing does help your body. Researchers have also shown that when people learn how to use humor, they cope better with stress. In fact, you don't actually have to be funny to get health benefits. Even if no one else rates you very high on your humor, the process of enjoying yourself or trying to change your attitude by thinking about things that disturb you from a humorous perspective can help.

Why work at adding humor to your life? For the pure relaxation that laughter brings (a sort of "internal jogging") and a refreshed outlook. Diabetes-wise humor serves as a social lubricant for difficult situations, enables you to talk about fears or anger stemming from diagnosis and management, prevents burnout from the chronic care of diabetes, builds self-esteem, and paradoxically, helps you face—not deny—the seriousness of diabetes. Mark Gorkin, a therapist and stand-up comic called the Stress Doc, reminds us to "practice safe stress and seek the higher power of humor: May the farce by with you."

A "FUN-TIONAL" GUIDE TO PHYSICAL FITNESS

Here's one way to get started on an exercise program.

1. Have a fit (Foreplay). Take the time to complain about why you don't wanna do it, moan how tired you are, or complain that you have nothing to wear, look awful in exercise clothes, and have no exercise buddy. Say how distorted those mirrors at the gym are. Ramble on about how your blood glucose might drop if you do too much. (So test and eat or take less insulin). Now, exaggerate your complaints until even you can hear how silly they sound. This fit can be contained in a 15-minute period, or for the well practiced, even less. You might say it is equivalent to 15 minutes of foreplay. Just remember, don't get stuck in performing only the fit. You've exercised your feelings, your vocal chords, and your sense of humor. Always follow this with the real thing, exercising your body.

2. Get fit. Start moving. This is the time when your walking shoes are fit to be tied. You can be prepared to seize an opportunity by having your walking shoes and a

snack to prevent or treat low blood glucose with you at all times. Being in action is the fun part.

3. Afterplay. Fit means being firm and calm and satisfied. Exercise does this for every body, even yours. This is the time when you feel the pleasant glow of well-used muscles and balanced emotions. You can gloat, tell yourself how happy you are that you exercised, how impressed you are with your discipline, how you surely can and will keep your blood glucose normal. **(positive self-talk)** You cool down, check your blood glucose, and eat lots of calories. (Kidding about the last one.) And be aware that it can go lower than usual for up to 18 hours after you exercise. One reason is that your muscles just keep on burning calories, even at rest. That's the reason you want muscle instead of fat (not just so kids won't kick sand in your face).

Remember, exercise is a habit, a positive addiction, and a good friend to turn to when you are anxious, sad, insecure, or overwhelmed. (It's a better friend than a box of cookies.) Exercise lifts your mood, maybe by altering the chemical balance in your brain. It actually gives you a feeling of completion, mastery, and discipline. It acts as an antidepressant, and in some studies has had as good an effect as therapy or medication. Exercise leaves you feeling

- exhilarated
- exorcised (of bad feelings)
- energized

You do have more energy when you're done. You may also have a new direction, or at least enough oomph to continue on with your regular plan.

A "FUN-TIONAL" GUIDE TO FOOD

Here are 10 or so commandments of good eating.

1. Thou shalt not be impulsive. Plan ahead for extras or binges. (For example, I know I'll want junior mints at the movies, therefore, I will not have bread with dinner.) When you make choices that are not so helpful, keep your sense of humor. It's not the end of your meal plan, just a little detour.

2. Thou shalt have style while eating.

- Chew slowly.
- Consciously swallow before you take your next bite.
- Put your fork down before the next bite.
- Drink sips of non-caloric beverages between bites.
- Pause between bites. You might find that you are a good listener, or when your mouth is not full, a good conversationalist.

3. Thou shalt not eat with the lights off. Calories do count, even if no one (including you) is looking. They also count if you are standing up or eating with your fingers.

4. Thou wast not born with a silver spoon in your mouth. Don't put it there while you're cleaning up after a big meal. (That goes for fingers, too.)

5. Thou shalt have a bodyguard or helper when you are cooking or cleaning up after a meal. Being left to clean up is lonely and dangerous. It could also signify that you may be spoiling your family or old-fashioned, thinking you have to do it all. Blood glucose is not as likely to rise when you prepare food or clean up with a family member or friend. (They do rise when you clean up by putting leftover food into you.)

6. Thou may chew sugarfree gum while cooking or clearing so as not to taste every dish too often. (Check with your dentist on this one.)

7. Thou shalt not eat everything on your plate. Leaving some food is a sign of being wealthy. As for the other leftovers from the meal, be a gracious hostess and give your company food to take home.

8. Thou shalt mind your peas and cues—the people, places, or things that trigger you to eat.

- Keep problem foods out of sight and stored in opaque containers.
- Unscrew the lightbulb in the refrigerator. If you don't see it, you are less likely to want it.
- Eat in the same place everyday—at the kitchen or dining-room table. Bedrooms and in front of the TV are for other things.
- Avoid buffets if you can, but once there, use a small plate and try to sit down and eat with a fork and a knife.
- When you are furious at someone and don't have the nerve to tell them, don't overeat. Write an imaginary letter to them; tell someone else about it; exercise (but for goodness sake, don't kick the dog).

9. Thou shalt remember that there is more to life than food. What other sources of pleasure or distraction do you have?

10. Thou shalt be a sensuous and sensible shopper. Shop for fresh and varied foods on a full stomach. Buy only what is on your list. Dress up when you shop so you feel relaxed and attractive. Think thin and healthy as you glide down the aisles. Pay attention to prices and people, not gingerbread cookies dancing in your head or in your hand.

11. Thou shalt think through decisions about eating. Be aware of what you eat (write it down), how much you eat, where you eat, with whom you eat, and the reason you're eating. Remember that blaming other people or circumstances for your behavior means that you are trying to give up control of your own life. First of all, you can't. It is inaccurate to blame, and second, it is a cop-out. Take 5 deep breaths before you make one false move. Think about 3 things:

- What prompted you to want to eat? **(past)**
- How long will it satisfy you in the **present?**
- Think about how you will feel after. **(future)**

Hint: High blood glucose makes you sleepy, weepy, and needing to pee—with a helping of guilt on top.

12. Thou shalt not deprive yourself—of good moments, of meaning in your life besides food and diabetes, and of fruits and vegetables. (Forgive my need to be concrete.)

13. This can be a lucky number. Thou shalt remember it takes 21 days to make a good habit. At that point, we are in the zone—an enlightened place where being good to ourselves does not take so much effort. Before this time, we often zone out by procrastination and avoiding making good choices.

HAVE FUN

Debbie Singer, a young woman with diabetes for 24 years, says: "Now, do I get mad at the person butting in about my diabetes? No, I first laugh at my own response, then I sit back for a moment and try to appreciate the curious nature of all human beings. I know that there is no spite in the question, rather there is concern. Not everyone can claim to have others concerned about them. Hey, I just found a benefit of hav-

ing diabetes." The process of taking time to form her perspective with humor helps her relax and is a positive buffer against negative thoughts and interactions.

Again, diabetes is not funny. Don't let it get you twice by taking away your sense of humor. Keep laughing. The life you save may be your own.

MY UNFAVORITE THINGS

(Sung to the tune of "My Favorite Things" from *The Sound of Music)*

Anger, anxiety, boredom, and guilt
Loneliness, emptiness
up to the hilt.
Frustration, sadness
such "tsouris" this brings
These are a few of my unfavorite things...

When the dog bites,
When the bee stings,
When I'm feeling sad,
I always remember these unfavorite things
and continue to feel so bad.

But then I remember
a new way of coping,
which brings me more pleasure
and brings me more hoping
and suddenly I know that happiness can be earned
by applying the principles of all that I have learned.

When the dog bites,
When the bee stings,
When I'm feeling sad,
I'll always remember these principle things
and then I won't feel so bad.

Resources

American Association for Marriage and Family Therapy
1133 15th Street NW, Suite 300
Washington, DC 20036
(202) 452-0109
(800) 374-2638
(202) 223-2329

American Association of Sex Educators, Counselors, and Therapists
P.O. Box 238
Mount Vernon, IA 52314-0238
For a list of certified sex therapists, send a business-size, self-addressed, stamped envelope.

American Psychiatric Association
1400 K Street, NW
Washington, D.C. 20005
(202) 682-6000

American Psychiatric Nurses Association
1200 19th Street, NW
Washington, D.C. 20036-2422
(202) 857-1133

American Psychological Association
750 1st Street, NE
Washington, DC 20002-4242
(202) 336-5500
(800) 374-2721

Council on Behavioral Medicine and Psychology
American Diabetes Association, Professional Section
1660 Duke Street
Alexandria, VA 22314
(800) 232-3472
http://www.diabetes.org

National Association of Social Workers
750 First Street NE, Suite 700
Washington, DC 20002
(202) 408-8600
(800) 638-8799

National Mental Health Association
(800) 969-NMHA (6642)
http://www.nmha.org

Neuro-Linguistic Programming
NLP Comprehensive
4895 Riverbend Rd., Suite A
Boulder, CO 80301
(303) 442-1102
(800) 233-1657
fax: (303) 442-0609

Siblings for Significant Change
823 United Nations Plaza, Room 808
New York, NY 10017
(212) 420-0776

Society of Behavioral Medicine
401 E. Jefferson Street, Suite 205
Baltimore, MD 20850-2617
(410) 251-2790

Society of Pediatric Psychology
c/o Donald Wertlieb, PhD, President
Eliot-Pearson Dept. of Child Study
Tufts University
Medford, MA 02155
(617) 627-3355
http://129.171.43.143/spp/

Stepfamily Association
#212 Lincoln Center
215 S. Centennial Mall
Lincoln, NE 68508

The Well Spouse Foundation
P.O. Box 801
New York, NY 10023
(212) 644-1241
(800) 838-0879
http://nhic-nt.health.org/htm/gen/htm/gen.exe/

EATING DISORDERS

American Anorexia/Bulimia Association
Suite 1R
293 Central Park West
New York, NY 10024
(212) 575-6200
http://members.aol.com/amanbu

National Association of Anorexia Nervosa and Associated Disorders
P.O. Box 7
Highland Park, IL 60035
(847) 831-3438
http://www.healthtouch.com/level1/leaflets/102952/102952.htm

National Institute of Mental Health
Eating Disorders Website
http://www.nimh.nih.gov/publicat/eatdis.htm

Depressed Anonymous
An international 12-step organization inspired by a woman who suffered from heart disease and depression. Offers local support groups for depression. For free information, call (502) 569-1989; send a SASE to Depressed Anonymous
P.O. Box 17471
Louisville, KY 40217
e-mail: depanon@ka.net

Emotions Anonymous
An international organization with more than 1,000 chapters. Fellowship for people experiencing emotional difficulties. Uses the 12-step program sharing experience, strength, and hopes to improve emotional health. Correspondence program for those who cannot attend meetings. Contact: Emotions Anonymous
P.O. Box 4245
St. Paul, MN 55104-0245
(612) 647-9712

Weight Watchers
(800) 651-6000

Overeaters Anonymous Headquarters
World Service Office
6075 Zenith Court, NE
Rio Rancho, NM 87124
(508) 891-2664
http://www.overeatersanonymous.org

Humor Project
10 Spring Street
Saratoga Springs, NY 12866
(518) 587-8770
magazine, resources, research

ABOUT THE AMERICAN DIABETES ASSOCIATION

The American Diabetes Association is the nation's leading voluntary health organization supporting diabetes research, information, and advocacy. Founded in 1940, the Association provides services to communities across the country. Its mission is to prevent and cure diabetes and to improve the lives of all people affected by diabetes.

For more than 50 years, the American Diabetes Association has been the leading publisher of comprehensive diabetes information for people with diabetes and the health care professionals who treat them. Its huge library of practical and authoritative books for people with diabetes covers every aspect of self care—cooking and nutrition, fitness, weight control, medications, complications, emotional issues, and general self care. The Association also publishes books and medical treatment guides for physicians and other health care professionals.

Membership in the Association is available to health care professionals and people with diabetes and includes subscriptions to one or more of the Association's periodicals. People with diabetes receive *Diabetes Forecast,* the nation's leading health and wellness magazine for people with diabetes. Health care professionals receive one or more of the Association's five scientific and medical journals.

For more information, please call toll-free:

Questions about diabetes: 1-800-DIABETES
Membership, people with diabetes: 1-800-806-7801
Membership, health professionals: 1-800-232-3472
Free catalog of ADA books: 1-800-232-6733
Visit us on the Web: www.diabetes.org
Visit us at our Web bookstore: merchant.diabetes.org